2·22·80

guide to
CROSS-COUNTRY SKIING

the
physician
and
sportsmedicine

guide to
CROSS-COUNTRY SKIING

EDWARD G. HIXSON, M.D.

SERIES EDITOR, PAUL SCHULTZ

McGRAW-HILL BOOK COMPANY

NEW YORK   ST. LOUIS   SAN FRANCISCO   DÜSSELDORF
LONDON   MEXICO   SYDNEY   TORONTO

1234567890MUMU876543210

LIBRARY OF CONGRESS CATALOGING IN PUBLICATION DATA
Hixson, Edward G
   The Physician and sportsmedicine guide to cross-country skiing.
   Includes index.
   1. Cross-country skiing—Physiological aspects.
2. Cross-country skiing—Accidents and injuries.
3. Physical fitness.   I. Physician and sportsmedicine.   II. Title.
RC1220.C77H59   617′.1027   79–21863
ISBN 0–07–029057–1

Illustrations by Elton Hoff.

Book design by Marsha Picker.

acknowledgments

2093185

THIS BOOK could not have been written without the cooperation of many colleagues. In Part 1, Advances in Cross-Country Skiing, Chapter 1, "Extending Your Knowledge of Cross-Country Skiing," was written in collaboration with Martha Roth and Thomas Jacobs, president of Reliable Racing Supply, Glens Falls, New York. Chapter 2, "Effective Cross-Country Skiing Technique," depends heavily on the work of Charles J. Dillman, Ph.D., associate professor of physical education and director of the Biomechanics Research Laboratory at the University of Illinois, Champaign-Urbana, and his research assistants Daniel M. India and Philip E. Martin. Their colleagues, C. H. Terry Ward, Keith French, Robert DaGiau, and Peter Davis, gave technical assistance in the filming of the work from which biomechanical analyses were made, and the project was supported by the U.S. Nordic Ski Team, John Bower, director; Dr. Francis B. Trudeau of Saranac Lake, New York; and Tony Wise, owner of Telemark Lodge in Cable, Minnesota. Dr. Dillman serves as Coordinator of Sports Medicine for the U.S. Ski Team (USST).

The sports psychology section of Chapter 2 draws on the work of Richard M. Suinn, Ph.D., professor and head of the Department of Psychology at Colorado State University, Fort Collins.

In Part 2, Training, Chapter 3, "A Training Program for Serious Cross-Country Skiers," is based on the work of Jim Page, of the USST staff, and Ulf Bergh, prominent Swedish sports physiologist and author of *Cross-Country Skiing*. Chapters 4 and 5, "Neuromuscular Training for Strength and Power" and "Training for Coordination, Balance, Agility, Flexibility, and Relaxation," are also based on Jim Page's work on a core training program for Olympic skiers. Chapter 5 also includes a stretching program used by Art Dickinson, trainer for the USST, and a relaxation routine developed by Dr. Richard Suinn and his colleagues at the University of Colorado as part of their work in sports psychology. Chapter 6, "Nutrition for Nordic Skiers," is based on the work of Art Dickinson and his colleague Emily Haymes, Ph.D.

In Part 3, Nordic Sports Medicine, Chapter 7, "Preventing Nordic Skiing Injuries," includes the work of Francis B. Trudeau, M.D., on skiers' common medical problems and on health prerequisites for Nordic competition. For the material in Chapter 9, "Who Looks Out for Nordic Skiers?" I must thank John Bower, director of the USST Nordic Program, and Steve Detwiler, leader of the Mount Van Hoevenberg Nordic Patrol.

Additional thanks to Dr. Robert B. Arnot, Dr. Robert Obma, Geoffrey Tesch, and Philip T. Wilson.

All of the above are united with the common goal of medicine and science in support of skiing.

EDWARD G. HIXSON, M.D., F.A.C.S.
Director
United States Nordic Ski Team
Medical Supervisory Team

contents

Introduction

WHY SHOULD you want to read another book about cross-country skiing? Hasn't it been promoted in this country as a do-it-yourself sport, and as the inexpensive winter recreational activity in contrast to the expensive one, downhill skiing? Haven't you heard that it is an activity on skis that you can walk away from without crutches? If you have read or heard these things and are thinking about taking up the sport, or if you have already been involved and have found that it is not quite as simple as you thought, then you should read this book.

The basis for this book is the manual prepared by Dr. Hixson and his associates for the U.S. National Nordic Ski Team. It has been adapted so that it may be useful for both the recreational and the competitive skier. No matter what your experience in this sport may have been, this book can help you achieve more effective and more enjoyable, as well as safer, skiing.

ALLAN J. RYAN, M.D., EDITOR-IN-CHIEF
The Physician and Sportsmedicine

one

ADVANCES IN CROSS-COUNTRY SKIING

1.
extending
your
knowledge of
cross-country
skiing

THIS BOOK is different. Most books on cross-country skiing begin with the same information: how the Scandinavians have been traveling on skis for at least four thousand years; how archaeologists have found well-preserved Stone Age skis in a Swedish peat bog; how the Byzantine historian Procopius described Finns "gliding" on what must have been skis; how medieval Scandinavian knights held ski tourneys.

When they get to the New World, all the cross-country skiing books describe how skiing began in America with the legendary "Snowshoe" Thompson, who delivered mail to the mining camps of the Sierra Nevada on skis in the 1840s, and who introduced ski touring to the towns he passed by. Then they go on to describe the pleasures of Nordic skiing, its many advantages over Alpine skiing, the splendid efforts of John Caldwell and other Olympic racers to popularize the sport, and Bill Koch's silver medal in the 1976 Innsbruck Olympics, the first time an American ever medaled in a cross-country event.

But we assume that you have read at least some of those books; that you are a serious cross-country skier who doesn't need to be coaxed. Your motive for reading this book, we think, is to learn how the Olympic racers train and how you can adapt their programs for your own use.

You won't find a discussion of cross-country technique in this book. We assume you have already mastered the diagonal stride, double-poling, the telemark turn, the snowplow, herringboning, the controlled fall. There are also no discussions of ski jumping, which really lies outside our scope, or of ski mountaineering, except in terms of exposure risks.

The basis of this material is the training, care, and feeding of cross-country ski racers. In the words of John Caldwell, the former Olympic skier and coach who is director of the National Hiking and Ski Touring Association, "The racing crowd generally sets the styles." In any sport, the most highly visible athletes are the most interesting; also, in purely practical terms, sports medicine research is generally done on them.

Although we will not be discussing technique, you should know that the racing form is the most efficient method of skiing. Almost everything that is said about cross-country ski racing is applicable to ski touring.

"Citizens' races" are becoming a popular winter feature of most snow-belt communities in the United States, where

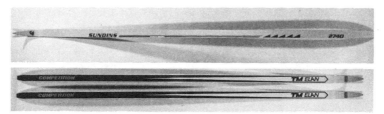

figure 1 Cross-country racing ski. Sundins model 2740. Air-channeled wood core. Plasticized sidewalls. Soft camber for young racers. (Courtesy of Reliable Racing Supply, Glens Falls, N.Y.)

figure 2 Cross-country racing skis. Elan model RB-SR. Air-channeled acrylic foam core with balsam and poplar wood. Sidewalls routed underfoot. Touring skis are cambered softer and are somewhat wider. (Courtesy of Reliable Racing Supply, Glens Falls, N.Y.)

more than 2 million recreational cross-country skiers live. You already know the difference between racing skis and touring skis (see Figures 1 and 2). You know the advantages and disadvantages of fishscales, mohair strips, other no-wax bottoms, and the various waxes and klisters.

You probably also know that at least twenty importers of cross-country equipment, as well as some American manufacturers, provide the serious skier with an excellent selection of skis, bindings, poles, boots, and waxes. Some large dealers, like Reliable Racing Supply of Glens Falls, New York, also carry track-setting equipment, timing systems, fencing, and all the associated paraphernalia of racing.

Roller skis and accessories—poles, brakes, gloves—are also available from cross-country equipment dealers, as are such refinements of the training program as the arm-and-shoulder-training "Exer-Genie,' and a mini-gym with different settings.

Skis

Wood bottoms, once upon a time, were cheaper and easier to maintain than glass fiber or other synthetic materials, and it used to be true that wax adhered to them better. Some racers still prefer laminated all-wood skis; they feel that plastic, glass fiber, and metal do not have the camber and flexibility of a well-made wood ski. But wooden skis are rapidly becoming artifacts of the past.

Most racers nowadays like the extra strength and lightness of the newer, foam-cored, glass fiber skis, some of them weighing less than 3 pounds. For glass fiber bottoms, hot-waxed paraffin seems to be the preferred method of waxing, a thin layer over the whole ski. Many racers like to use a "kicker" wax right under the foot, and some also use a "glider" at tip and tail.

Waxing, however, is such an idiosyncratic matter that it is impossible to give any general advice about it in a book, except to say that it is probably advisable to stick with one set, or system, of waxes, at least until one is very familiar with one's own performance, and with the behavior of one's skis, in different kinds of snow. Most experienced skiers use highly individual mixtures.

Boots and Clothes

In general, the best racing boot is the lightest and most flexible, and the best clothes are the least bulky or confining. Many boots these days are molded of plastic or foam. They are cheaper, but most racers prefer leather, which is warmer, longer-lasting, and more flexible. (Figure 3)

It is fashionable for racers to wear sleek one-piece suits of synthetic materials; they weigh only a few ounces and offer no wind resistance, but they are expensive and give almost no protection against the cold. Your choice of clothing should be influenced by the weather, how long you are going to be exposed to it, and whether you can

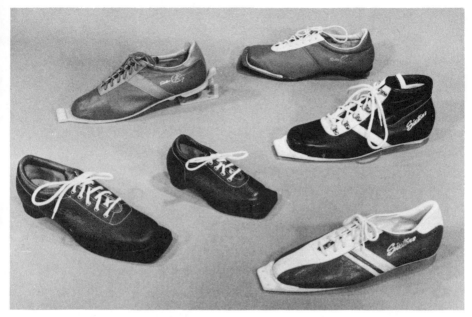

figure 3 Cross-country racing boots in different styles and sizes. These are made by sixtens from goat or cow hides. (Courtesy of Reliable Racing Supply, Glens Falls, N.Y.)

reasonably expect to change as soon as the race is finished. Racers are usually wet with perspiration at the end of a race, and nylon or acrylic fiber clothing will not permit the moisture to evaporate.

Cotton mesh underthings (thermal underwear for really cold days, below 0°F) and layers of cotton flannel or thin wool shirts, with woolen knickers and knee socks, make the best cross-country ski clothing. Many skiers swear by wool because it stays warm even when wet. Thin cotton or silk socks under your woolen knee socks will protect your feet against excessive sweating by conducting moisture away from the skin.

Gloves

Racing gloves and low, thin boots are not proper attire for long training in very cold weather. Insulated touring boots, or gaiters worn over your racing boots, will protect your feet. Alpine gloves will protect your hands. Some skiers prefer mittens, which are warmer than gloves, but many racers find that even awkward gloves give better control.

Poles

Glass fiber or aluminum poles, light and practically unbreakable, are best for racing. For regular ski touring, some skiers prefer bamboo because of its low cost and springiness. The newest, lightest poles (and also the most expensive) are made of carbon fiber, which is very strong and quite stiff (Figure 4). Serious skiers can switch pole tips, using carbide tips for icy tracks and conventional steel tips for softer snow. Roller-skiing requires use of elastic carbide tips.

Racing poles have lightweight, narrow baskets because they are used on packed tracks. For touring in deeper snow, ski poles should have a wider basket, to give you some push. Canted baskets are sometimes thought to increase speed (see Figure 4, second and third from the left). Leather or cork pole grips are really the best; most of the new poles can be bought with leather grips. Straps should be made of leather also.

Bindings

Pin bindings are still standard, although pinless spring bindings are always available (Figure 5). Some racers prefer

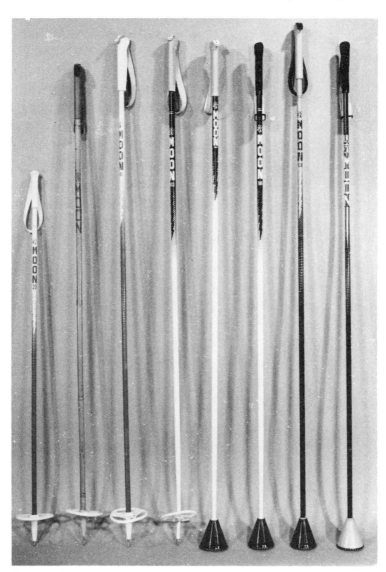

figure 4 Cross-country ski poles. The four on the left have steel tips; those on the right, tips of elastic carbide. Note the canted baskets, second and third from the left. Some have carbon fiber and others aluminum shafts. (Courtesy of Reliable Racing Supply, Glens Falls, N.Y.)

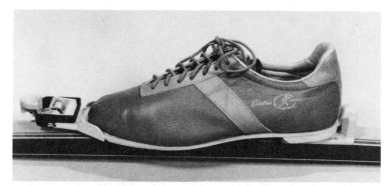

figure 5 Light metal, spring-loaded, pinless bindings. (Courtesy of Reliable Racing Supply, Glens Falls, N.Y.)

the pinless kind for rough terrain because there is no risk of losing pins and less risk of tearing off boot soles.

The choice of gear is up to you, and ultimately, of course, it matters less than your attitude and training. This book will introduce you to a little serious sports physiology, a rigorous training program, and the rudiments of Nordic sports medicine. Because your sport combines the greatest strength and the greatest endurance of any athletic event, Nordic racers are held up as heroic models—and not just by sports physiologists.

2.
effective
cross-country
skiing
technique

Biomechanical Determinations

THE BIOMECHANICS of sports is a relatively young field that uses the science of mechanics to analyze sports performance. In the study of sports techniques, the principles and methods of mechanics are used to describe and evaluate selected motion and force parameters of performance. The goal of this research is to provide a scientific basis for improving sports performance.

The first procedure in biomechanical study is the making of a scientific record of the skill to be analyzed, usually with high-speed 16mm film at frame rates between 100 and 200 frames per second. Filming procedure is strictly controlled. The films are then analyzed by an electronic digitizer linked to a computer.

The biomechanical investigator's aim is to isolate the critical mechanical factors in performance. The descriptive data for a given population—in this case, serious cross-country skiers—are evaluated by mechanical and statistical methods. Practical performance guidelines based on these evaluations can provide the coach, teacher, or skier with specific information about the best way to perform a given skill.

Only a few biomechanical investigations of cross-country skiing have been conducted, most of them concerned with the diagonal stride. Four recent studies, two Swiss, one Swedish, and one from the University of Illinois, provide the information for the following analysis.

From a mechanical viewpoint, the performance objective of cross-country skiing is *velocity*. Every competitive cross-country skier is trying to maintain velocity from stride to stride. The higher the average rate of movement, the better the performance. This is the first step in biomechanical analysis: formulation of the objective.

The next step is to determine what mechanical aspects of the skill, such as force or motion, directly influence the objective. For a cyclical activity like cross-country skiing, an equation of performance has been derived that relates two performance factors to the objective, velocity:

$$\text{Velocity} = \text{Stride Length (SL)} \times \text{Stride Rate (SR)}$$

The equation states that the average rate of velocity of a skier, per cycle of movement (stride), is a product of the distance moved (stride length) and the rate at which the basic cycle is repeated per second (stride rate). A cross-country skier who wishes to improve performance must in-

SL = 2.88 m (9.45 ft)
STRIDE T = .620 s
SR = 1.61 strides/s
    (97 strides/min)

$V = SL \bullet SR$
4.64 m/s = 2.88 m   1.61 str/s
(10.4 miles/hr)

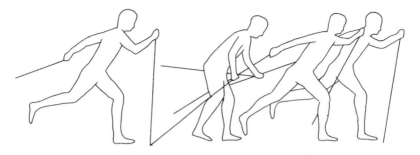

figure 1 Stride length and rate for highly skilled skier

crease the average rate of movement over ground. This can be accomplished by increasing the length of the stride, which is the basic unit of movement in cross-country skiing, or the rate of striding, or both.

Figure 1 illustrates the application of the stride length-rate equation. This particular sequence starts when the right pole is inserted into the snow (A) and terminates when the left pole enters the snow (D). From A to B, the body is moved along primarily on the supporting left ski by the thrust action of the right arm. At B, the supporting ski becomes stationary and the body swings forward over this base of support, generating a thrust, or kick, by the support leg onto the opposite ski. From C to D, the body glides along on the new supporting right ski until the opposite left pole is planted (D). After this glide, the sequence occurs again, with the opposite leg and arm. It is the repetition of this basic unit of movement—pole-in to pole-in equals one step or stride—that propels the skier over the snow.

The total horizontal distance moved by the body from A to D is the length of the stride. Film analysis of the highly skilled skier in Figure 1 showed a stride length of 2.88 meters (m), or 9.45 feet. The time taken to cover this distance was .62 seconds. Thus, in one second, this skier completed 1.61 strides. This skier's stride rate can be computed at 1.61 strides per second, or 97 strides per minute. The velocity of the skier in Figure 1 can now be calculated by the performance equation:

$$V = SL \times SR$$
$$V = 2.88 \text{ m} \times 1.61 \text{ strides/sec}$$
$$V = 4.64 \text{ m/sec, or } 10.4 \text{ mph}$$

The average stride velocity for this skier, 10.4 miles per hour, is a typical speed in the diagonal stride for a skilled skier. A skier who continues at this pace will cover 4.64 meters, or 15.3 feet, of ground for every second of skiing. But what is important is that we now have a description of how the skilled skier attains this speed: he travels at a velocity of 10.4 miles per hour by covering 2.88 meters in each stride and repeating 1.6 strides every second.

Figure 2 is a diagram of the cross-country stride, pole plant left to pole plant right, for an average skier. Comparative analysis of the highly skilled versus the average skier shows the following results:

	V	=	SL	×	SR
Skilled	4.64 mps		2.88 m		1.61 strides/sec
Average	3.51 mps		2.22 m		1.58 strides/sec
Difference	1.13 mps		.66 m		.03 strides/sec
	(2.50 mph)				

SL = 2.22 m (7.28 ft)
STRIDE T = .632 s
SR = 1.58 strides/s
    (95 strides/min)

$V = SL \bullet SR$
3.51 m/s = 2.22 m 1.58 str/s
(7.9 miles/hr)

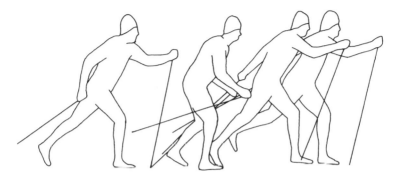

figure 2   Stride length and rate for average-skilled skier

The skilled skier goes 2.5 miles per hour faster primarily because of a longer stride length. The difference in stride rate accounts for a relatively small proportion of the difference in velocity. In general, the main cause of the differences in velocity between skilled and average skiers is the length of stride or the distance attained per stroke. An average skier who wants to travel faster should devote attention and training to increasing the distance per stroke, assuming that increases in distance can be obtained without a reduction in the stride rate. This is reasonable within the velocity range of 7 to 10 miles per hour.

Stride length seems to be more critical than stride rate for increasing velocity from 7 to 10 miles per hour. Some evidence suggests, however, that increases in velocity *above* 10 miles per hour in the diagonal stride, such as are attained by world-class skiers, may be a result of increases in stride rate. The data are variable, and in any case, few of

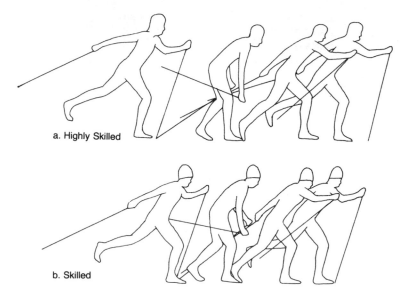

a. Highly Skilled

b. Skilled

figure 3 Comparison between high-skilled and skilled skiers in distance attained per stride (both illustrations on same scale)

even the most serious skiers will be working at this order of velocity.

Figure 3 further illustrates the difference in stride length between skiers at different skill levels. The skier shown at the top, *a*, of Figure 3 can be considered highly skilled. The skier at the bottom, *b*, is classed as skilled. Both skiers in Figure 3 have been drawn to the same scale to illustrate more clearly the differences in distance per stroke.

Both skiers have completed the same cycle of motion, pole plant left to pole plant right. The highly skilled skier traveled .58 centimeters (1.9 feet) farther than the skilled skier during the same cycle. The time of stride for the better skier was .548 seconds, while the other skier had a slightly faster time, .526 seconds. The difference in time per stride, 22 milliseconds, contributed much less to the difference in velocity between the two (10.5 miles per hour for the highly skilled, 8.5 miles per hour for the skilled) than stride length.

How can the average skier obtain more distance per stroke in the diagonal stride? The techniques that appear to contribute to a longer stride can be analyzed in relation to the three phases of the stride: the kick, the glide, and the pole implantation.

The Kick Phase. A more effective kick or a better use of the energy generated in this phase will increase distance per stride. Figure 4 traces the kick phase.

This phase, as defined in recent research, begins when both legs come together during the period when the sup-

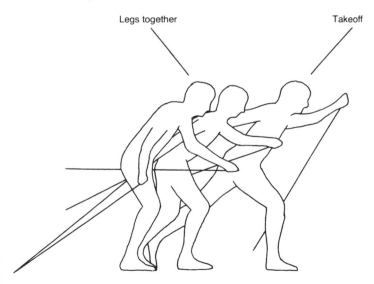

Legs together   Takeoff

figure 4 Sequence tracing of the kick phase

porting ski is stationary. Termination of the kick occurs when the thrusting leg is fully extended and the support ski begins to spring from the track.

Biomechanical research has shown that the *position of the body* at the initiation of the kick is one of the factors contributing to good thrust. Skilled skiers typically have a more flexed position, with the body weight farther forward, than poorer skiers. The angle of the trunk with the ski (Angle T in Figure 5) approaches 45 degrees. The lower leg is flexed forward to form an angle with the ski of about 60 degrees (Angle A). The body's mass is centered over the toes. Poorer skiers generally have a more upright trunk and a more nearly vertical lower leg (Angle A would approach 90 degrees), and their weight is centered over the ball or heel of the foot. A more flexed, forward-leaning position facilitates a direct forward application of force

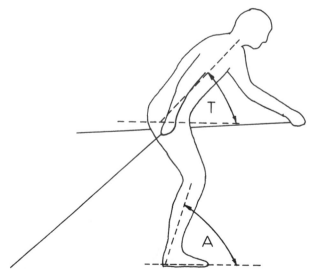

figure 5   Body position at initiation of kick

and provides for a quicker kick, characteristic of better skiers. This is how they get greater thrust in a shorter time.

Analysis of the kicking movements of expert skiers indicates that strong, *explosive muscles* are needed to generate a large force in a short time. Since no specific exercises have yet been developed that simulate the dynamic conditions of the kick, skiers must rely on their usual endurance training plus their genetic endowment for explosive power.

A third factor that might improve the kick is *conceptualization*. The objective of the kick is to generate a relatively small horizontal force to maintain or slightly increase the body's velocity as it swings forward over the stationary ski. However, to generate this force, the ski must be pressed vertically into the snow, and this requires a relatively large force. The maximum values for this vertical component are about 1.5 times body weight for the average touring skier and 3 times body weight for the cross-country racer.

This large normal force, perpendicular to the skiing surface, is produced by the vigorous upward acceleration of all body segments involved in the kick. Perhaps conceptualizing the kick as a *vigorous extension* (to set the ski) and a *slight push* (to maintain and increase velocity) would help skiers improve this aspect of the stride.

A fourth factor that contributes to an effective kick is the correct use of body parts other than the legs to generate the kick force. Upward acceleration of any limbs increases the vertical load on the ski; thus, movement of the arms, one backward and up and the other forward and up, plus vigorous extension of the trunk, adds to the force pressing the ski into the snow.

Good skiers extend their trunks vigorously for a short

distance in the kick phase. This trunk extension usually begins at 45 degrees (see Angle T in Figure 5) and increases to about 55 degrees. The vigorous short extension, only 10 degrees, of the large mass of trunk can add significantly to the reaction force between ski and snow.

The Glide Phase. At the end of the kick, the skier begins a free glide on the opposite ski. Figure 6 illustrates this phase. The distance attained during the glide depends to a large extent on the effectiveness of the kick. For a good skier, this phase can account for at least 25 percent of the total stride distance. Technique can be adjusted, however, to optimize the kick force generated. A well-balanced body is important in increasing the distance during glide. Better skiers keep the rear ski farther back than poorer skiers. During the glide the trunk should remain stationary, with the

End of kick   Pole plant

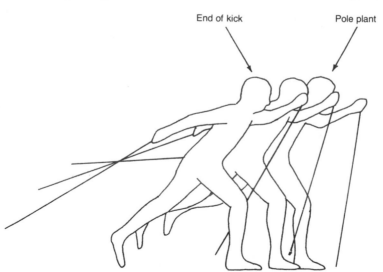

figure 6 Sequence drawings of the glide phase

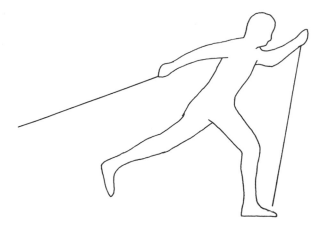

figure 7 Body position during glide for high-skilled skier

body weight slightly behind the ball of the foot. Figure 7 shows the sliding position of a highly skilled skier.

Pole Implantation Phase. The free glide ends when the pole is inserted into the snow. From this point, the skier rides on the support ski, moving along by a force generated by the shoulder-arm complex. The pole implantation phase ends when the support ski stops and the body begins to swing forward over the point of support in preparation for the kick. Figure 8 shows the sequence of body positions and arm-pole actions during this phase.

Biomechanical analysis has shown that it is the differences in distance attained during pole implantation that really distinguish better skiers from poorer ones. A range of 50 to 60 percent of the difference in stride length between highly skilled and average skiers occurs during this phase. Good skiers can travel 30 to 40 centimeters farther during this phase than average skiers.

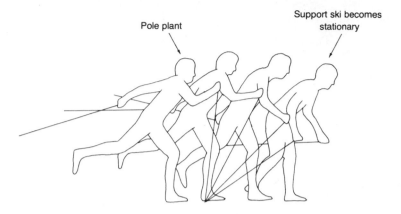

figure 8 Pole implantation phase

Pole-plant technique contributes to this difference. Figure 9 illustrates the contrast between the pole plant of a highly skilled skier (*top*) and that of a less skilled one (*bottom*). In general, better skiers plant the pole 15 to 25 centimeters farther in front of the supporting foot, with the pole in a more upright position. Their trunks are flexed forward more, and their elbows are more flexed when inserting the pole.

This pole plant also causes a different arm drive. Figure 9 shows the differences in arm action between highly skilled and skilled skiers. Better skiers coordinate their trunk movement with the bending of their arms more so than less skilled skiers. During pole implantation, highly skilled skiers flex the trunk and extend the upper arm from the shoulder, the forearm from the elbow, in a coordinated pattern. Less skilled skiers use a more continuous straight-arm push, extending only the shoulder muscles. The pattern of action of the highly skilled skier provides sequential application of force through a greater distance and is more effective.

Summary. Available biomechanical data show that average skilled cross-country skiers can improve their technique in the diagonal stride by increasing their distance per stroke. The following adjustments in the kick, glide, and pole implantation phases of the stride can help the average skier attain greater distance per stride.

KICK PHASE. Before the kick, when both legs are together, a flexed, forward-leaning position facilitates a quick thrust in

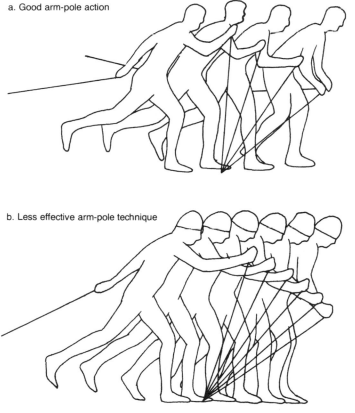

a. Good arm-pole action

b. Less effective arm-pole technique

figure 9 Comparison of arm-pole action

the direction of motion. Once the pattern of the diagonal stride has been established, the purpose of the kick is to maintain body velocity and increase momentum slightly. This action requires a relatively small force in the direction of motion, but to create this thrust, a relatively large force must press the supporting ski into the snow.

This large, perpendicular force is generated by the vigorous upward acceleration of all body segments involved in the kick. If the kick can be conceptualized as a vigorous *extension*, to set the ski, and a *slight push*, to maintain and increase body velocity, this aspect of the stride can be optimized for each skier. Better skiers generate a more effective thrust in a shorter time. Analysis of the kick reveals that power exercises, simulating the dynamic requirements of cross-country skiing, should complement the usual cardiorespiratory endurance training of cross-country skiers. Vigorous, brief extension of the trunk during the kick phase produces a more effective thrust.

GLIDE PHASE. A balanced body position, without compensating movements, facilitates the glide. There should be little movement of the trunk, and the body weight should be placed slightly behind the ball of the foot.

POLE IMPLANTATION PHASE. The greatest differences in distance per stride are noted during this phase, so it probably has the most potential for improvement. The average skier generally plants the pole close to or behind the foot, at an angle to the skiing surface, with a straight arm. Better skiers seem to coordinate the thrust, flexing the trunk and extending the upper arm and then the forearm. Average skiers should work on planting the pole a greater distance in front of the support foot and on maintaining a more erect position. The arm should be flexed at pole plant, and the trunk should lean forward.

two

TRAINING

The four chapters in this section are packed with information, all of which is based on work done with and for the U.S. Nordic Ski Team.

There may be more information here, in fact, than you care to know. Don't worry about skipping some of the suggestions for rigorous, year-round training activities. You can adjust some of the USST regimen to your own purposes, at whatever level you find yourself. Some of the data, especially in the Chapter 3 figures, refer to full-time competitive skiers. There's no need for you to feel chagrined if you can't match the training times of world-class Nordic ski racers.

We've included this information to show you what the outer limits of training are. But the tips on relaxation and diet can be useful to anybody, especially a serious recreational athlete like yourself. So read on—and keep some grains of salt handy.

3.
a training program for serious cross-country skiers

Energy Yield

YEAR-ROUND conditioning programs are necessary for any athlete who hopes to achieve high levels of performance. The best training, of course, is the sport itself. But good snow cover is limited, in most areas, to only three months each year. In order to improve, skiers must supplement skiing practice with dry-land exercises that duplicate skiing movements.

Cross-country skiing is one of the most physically demanding of sports. Skiers have to perform technically difficult maneuvers in a taxing physical environment. Top performance requires a sound physiological base and an intense conditioning program of activities that relates specifically to skiing.

There are three sets of activities that promote the efficient development of a skier's physiological base: (1) activities that increase energy yield, both aerobic and anaerobic, (2) neuromuscular activities that increase strength and power, and (3) activities that build coordination, balance, agility, flexibility, and relaxation.

A number of energy-yield activities, aerobic and anaerobic, will contribute to the efficient development of a skier's physiological base. The information in this chapter, and that in the two following, is not intended to outline a specific program for all skiers, but rather seeks to provide a factual basis for a sound program of dry-land training. Trainers of the U.S. Nordic Ski Team use this information to design their skiers' dry-land training programs, and these chapters are based on them.

Aerobic and Anaerobic Training. The body has two energy-producing or metabolic systems, aerobic and anaerobic. The *aerobic* system acts only in the presence of oxygen. In aerobic metabolism, glucose and fat are broken down and combined with oxygen to release energy. The aerobic system is efficient and will always be used when oxygen is available. Aerobic metabolism supplies all the body's energy requirements in the resting state.

Lung capacity—getting oxygen into the body—is an important determinant of aerobic efficiency. So is a healthy circulatory system, which effectively distributes to the tissues the oxygen that reaches the bloodstream in the lungs.

Aerobic Metabolism

Glucose
Fat $+$ Oxygen $=$ Body energy $+$ waste products $(CO_2) + H_2O$

The *anaerobic* system functions in the absence of oxygen. In anaerobic metabolism, glucose and fats are broken down directly. The aerobic system is slow to react to changes in the intensity and activity. When a skier needs a surge of power, the anaerobic system is called on as a source of quick energy. But its cost is great: the end product of anaerobic metabolism is *lactic acid*, which can't be given off like the end products of aerobic metabolism, water and carbon dioxide. If lactic acid accumulates in the muscles, it causes fatigue and diminished performance. So the anaerobic system can function only for a maximum of two or three minutes.

Anaerobic Metabolism

Glucose + Calcium = Body energy + lactic acid + H_2O

The anaerobic, or quick-energy, system is the dominant source of energy for intense workouts of very short duration. For longer workouts, the aerobic system is called on. Here are the relative contributions of the two systems to bouts of exercise ranging from ten seconds to two hours:

Metabolic Contribution, Percent	10 sec	1 min	2 min	4 min	10 min	30 min	60 min	120 min
Anaerobic	85	65–70	50	30	10–15	5	2	1
Aerobic	15	30–35	50	70	85–90	95	98	99

Most of the energy for cross-country skiing comes from the aerobic metabolism. But the chart assumes that exertion stays at nearly the same level of intensity throughout the given period, and this is not accurate for skiers. More than any other sport, cross-country skiing involves varying levels of intensity and a work load that shifts intricately between the aerobic and anaerobic systems.

The difficulty of calculating a skier's energy requirements is shown in Figure 1. This is a graph of part of a three-loop, cross-country race. The arrows at the bottom indicate changes in terrain direction. The lines at the top indicate changes in the skier's heart rate over this terrain. Maximum heart rate and maximum oxygen uptake are approached and even exceeded several times.

Skiers must maintain performance at a high level during sudden changes in intensity. The way to maintain high-level performance is to supply as much oxygen as possible for aerobic work and to develop tolerance to anaerobic conditions for those times when it is necessary to go into oxygen debt.

Cardiovascular Needs. A cross-country skier needs (1) a high maximum oxygen capacity, abbreviated Max VO_2,

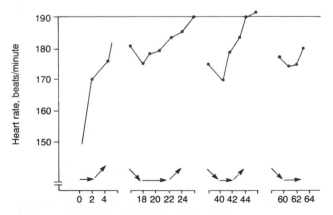

figure 1   Heart rate of a skier during a 21-km race (3 loops of 7 km)

Place (average)

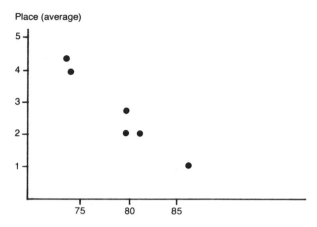

figure 2 Max VO₂, milliliters per kilogram of body weight

and (2) the ability to perform for long periods at a high percentage of that capacity. This second need is called a *high anaerobic threshold*; the skier's goal is to consume as much oxygen as possible so as to avoid using the anaerobic system and accumulating lactic acid.

A close relationship has been shown among top skiers between oxygen capacity and performance. In 1974, a Swedish investigative team identified the five most important competitions of the year and analyzed the performance of six of their best skiers in terms of their oxygen capacity (VO₂). Figure 2 summarizes their findings.

Oxygen capacity is determined to some extent by genetic inheritance; it can be improved by training, but only within certain limits. Fortunately, results are not always mathematically related, as they seem to be in Figure 2. Nonetheless, VO₂ is an important marker for the skier and should be developed to the highest possible level.

The second cardiovascular need for cross-country skiers is a high anaerobic threshold. This threshold is the level above which the anaerobic system dominates performance, and it is dramatically influenced by efficient training. Top skiers can operate for long periods at 80 to 90 percent of their maximum capacities without being seriously fatigued by lactic acid accumulation.

Training can raise the threshold. If a skier with a Max VO_2 of 80 milliliters per kilogram can tap 80 percent of his Max VO_2 for 30 kilometers, his projected time will be about 104 minutes; if he can tap 85 percent of his Max VO_2 for 30 kilometers, his projected time will be about 98 minutes; and if he can tap 85 percent of his Max VO_2 *and improve* his Max VO_2 by 5 percent, to 84 milliliters per kilogram, his projected time will be about 91 minutes.

Frank Shorter, the United States marathon runner, has achieved great success by being able to tap a very high percentage of his maximum capacity. His Max VO_2 is considered low in comparison with other world-class runners.

The way to increase Max VO_2 is to train at sufficient intensity so as to reach your maximum heart rate, or close to it. Energy spurts, however, involve the anaerobic system, and since anaerobic work leads to lactic acid accumulations and cannot be maintained for long periods, high and low intensities must be alternated.

The most efficient technique for achieving the high-intensity loading of the oxygen transport system necessary to improve Max VO_2 is *interval training*, or repeated anaerobic periods alternating with rest periods or periods of greatly reduced pace.

Interval training is most appropriate for cross-country skiers because the terrain makes Nordic skiing a sport of naturally varying intensities (see Figure 1). A great deal of ski-training exercise is called *natural interval training*, since a steady state of energy expenditure becomes impossible on the terrain.

Max VO₂ can be increased fairly quickly, so interval training doesn't have to go on throughout the year. About six weeks of interval training should come at the end of the dry-land training period, after a good endurance base of aerobic training has been established. Some anaerobic interval training is useful during the winter, a few weeks before major competition. Natural intervals are basic all year, but aerobic exercise should predominate; that is, your heart rate should be at or below your anaerobic threshold.

Increasing your capacity to tap a high percentage of your VO₂ will raise your anaerobic threshold. This is accomplished by *distance* or *endurance* activities. Long training near the anaerobic threshold increases your ability to endure prolonged work below the threshold. This activity can be done either at "steady-state" levels, with a relatively constant heart rate, or through natural interval exercise on uneven terrain, such as cross-country courses. This type of training makes up the major part of a good cross-country-skiing training program and must be done throughout the year. The desired training effect—raising the anaerobic threshold—seems more closely related to the amount of time spent training than to the type of exercise employed.

2093185

Planning a Year-Round Program. The Olympic training year is divided into three periods: (1) dry-land conditioning, (2) transition to snow, and (3) skiing (see Figure 3). There is a delicate balance involved in training: too little, at too low an intensity, will not produce the desired training effect. Too-high intensity, or too much training (or insufficient rest), will tear down a skier and block the accomplishment of training goals.

Training hours, kilometers, and intensities should be varied to allow skiers to build toward a winter peak and to

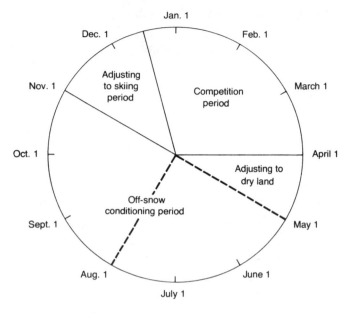

figure 3   U.S. Ski Team training year

insure the efficient development of energy output capacities. Figure 4 gives some guidelines for training amounts. Notice, however, that no figures are given for kilometers or hours, only percentages of the maximum, postulated in the November transition to snow. This permits any skier to adapt this guide, although it originally applied to full-time competitive skiers. Once you decide on your own yearly goals for total distance and hours, you can use this chart to figure each month's appropriate training.

Intensity is a more difficult concept to quantify. At low levels of intensity, work is done at a lower heart rate at more steady levels; there is less fluctuation in range. At higher levels, more natural interval work is done, with greater variations in heart rate.

APRIL TRANSITION TO DRY LAND. After the intensity of the winter, especially if it included competition, you should drop back significantly in the intensity and amount of training you do. This period is the end of one training year and the beginning of another. Your muscles will have to readjust gradually to running, biking, hiking, and roller-skiing. It is better not to plan rigid training schedules during April; train as the spirit moves you, as long as you are maintaining some quality activity. This is also the month to plan your training year.

APRIL–OCTOBER. The most important objective of this period is to build a base that will enable you to handle the long, intense winter, whether you ski competitively or not. In general, it is best to begin with longer, less intense workouts in the spring and work toward shorter, more intense workouts in September and October.

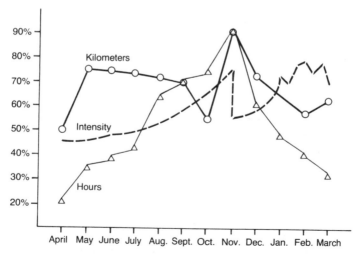

figure 4 Monthly training amounts for full-time skiers

Strength training, besides the normal increments developed by hiking or roller-skiing, should be emphasized, if necessary, from May through August. Gains in strength can then be maintained for the rest of the dry-land period.

Interval training is best combined with an increasingly intense endurance program in September and October. Six to eight weeks of intervals should suffice for maximum gains in speed and power for cross-country skiing. During the rest of the dry-land period, intervals should be done only enough to keep the muscles acquainted with them.

NOVEMBER–DECEMBER. On-snow training begins. This period will vary according to the availability of snow. In any case, the cross-country athlete should duplicate, in six to eight weeks, the rhythm of training done over the previous six months; begin with long, slow workouts and end with faster, somewhat shorter ones. The intensity of your workouts is important; use Figures 3, 4, and 5 to help you figure the appropriate amounts and intensities.

JANUARY–MARCH. These are the months of actual skiing and competition for most cross-country skiers. In general, the important races come in February and March, though there are local variations. January can be a time of mixed medium-distance and interval training and adjustment to racing. Some racing is important in December as well, although early results shouldn't be taken seriously. Many starts are needed for a skier to reach racing stride.

The amount and intensity of training should be reduced just before important competitions. Especially for young racers, a break in amount and intensity may be appropriate in the middle of a long competition season.

The U.S. Ski Team energy-yield training program consists of running, roller-skiing, hiking, and biking, as well as skiing. Most of the training is distance or endurance training, with some interval work mixed in. Figure 5 shows the approximate annual distribution of training activities.

Endurance Training. Since the aim of distance training is the development of aerobic endurance, each of these activities is done in such a way as to maximize its aerobic effects.

RUNNING. Some running can be done at a steady pace, with a constant heart rate, but the best form of distance running for ski training is *natural intervals*, continuous running for 45 to 120 minutes over hilly terrain. This type of workout most closely simulates the energy demands of skiing. A good gauge for intensity is to approach 85 to 100 percent of your maximum heart rate on uphills, 60 percent on downhills, and 70 to 80 percent on the flat.

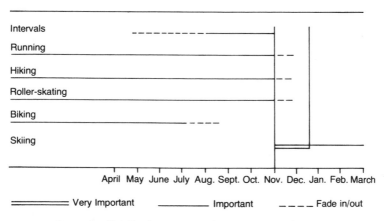

figure 5 Relative importance of training activities

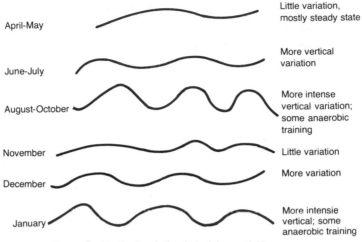

figure 6 Vertical variation in training activities

The amount of vertical variation should increase steadily throughout the six-month basic conditioning period and then during the six- to eight-week period of transition to snow (see Figure 6).

ROLLER-SKIING. Roller-skiing can be the most specific form of dry-land exercise for cross-country skiers. However, young skiers may find it has a negative effect on their technique unless they are already accomplished snow skiers.

Roller-skiing can load the oxygen transport system maximally, and during prolonged work on roller skis, lactic acid levels are lower at a certain percentage of Max VO_2. The oxygen transport system therefore develops more here than during running, with enhancement of aerobic power and endurance.

Like running, roller-skiing is best done on uneven terrain. Continuous natural interval training is recommended. Workouts can vary from one to three hours. Use the diagonal technique only on uphill slopes; double-poling is the proper roller-ski technique on the flat. Be careful on downhill sections. If possible, have someone along in a car with tools, bandages, water, and room for you if you should injure yourself.

HIKING. Speed hiking or mountain running is excellent energy-yield training. A good speed hike once a week for two to four hours is a healthy endurance workout. The main advantage, besides the psychological lift of a day in the mountains, is that hiking exaggerates the ups and downs of the hilly terrain.

Uphill hiking really gives the oxygen transport system a workout. Your heart rate may increase to its maximum on uphills, whereas hiking on the flat produces only about 80 percent of the maximum. Hiking also involves prolonged work at a high percentage of Max VO_2 and increases tolerance to lactic acid concentrations.

If you're fortunate enough to live near the mountains, you're undoubtedly familiar with their sudden weather changes. But if you're hiking in the mountains on a trip, be sure to wear proper hiking shoes and socks and to carry adequate clothing.

BIKING. Biking is a good way to accumulate kilometers at a lower intensity and in a shorter time than other forms of distance training offer. Uneven or hilly terrain, again, is best. You may find you want to phase out biking as part of your training after July if your program demands more intensity than a normal biking workout provides.

SKIING. Skiing is, of course, the best form of distance exercise. Olympic trainers currently believe that as soon as the transition to skiing has been made, no other form of training is necessary unless the weather makes skiing impossible. When you first get back on the snow, flat-terrain sessions are best because they allow you to adjust your technique. As the transition to snow continues, you can seek out more uneven terrain for natural interval training.

OTHER DISTANCE TRAINING. Effective forms of distance training include rowing, running with poles (a technique adapted from the Scandinavians), kayaking, and even enduro motorcycle riding. The most important criterion for distance training is whether it enhances aerobic power and endurance.

Interval Training. The objective of interval training is to increase both Max VO_2 and lactic acid tolerance. Interval training allows you to load your oxygen transport system beyond the demands of continuous training. Rest periods permit lactic acid concentrations to dissipate, so you can return to high-intensity levels for more repetitions. Interval work has proved to be the most effective way to increase oxygen uptake, enlarge oxygen transport, and develop tolerance to lactate concentrations in the blood.

Unlike aerobic training, which involves a long-term program, the goals of a good interval program can be accomplished in six to eight weeks. And since interval training is high-intensity, it also provides good pace training. Race-pace and greater-than-race-pace training will improve your tempo and speed of movement, and for this reason it's desirable to do interval work during the competition season.

However, during natural interval and interval training, you don't need to push the pace. Your optimum speed is the lowest speed at which your oxygen transport system is maximally loaded. Your heart rate should be about ten beats below your maximum at the end of each interval workout.

	Work Periods	Rest Periods	Repetitions
Long Intervals	2–10 minutes	2–5 minutes	3–10
Short Intervals	60–90 seconds	20–30 seconds	10–30
Very Short Intervals	10–20 seconds	5–15 seconds	20–60 minutes
Natural Intervals	Continuous running for 45–120 minutes in hilly terrain		

During rest intervals, your heart rate should recover to around 125 beats per minute. You can make a simple six-second pulse check immediately after work intervals and at the end of rest periods (multiplying your six-second pulse rate times 10 gives you your heart rate per minute).

Rest periods can be either active or passive. Jogging during rest intervals will prevent the lactic acid from clearing completely and can lead to increased tolerance. Passive rest, like sitting or stretching, allows complete lactic-acid clearing and leads to improvement in the Max VO_2. Both types of rest should be used alternately.

Be careful to individualize your interval training. Sometimes an athlete trains too hard and doesn't recover between work intervals. Don't resume work until your heart rate drops to 125, at most. If your heart rate doesn't recover within the rest interval, quit your workout for that day.

Interval training can be done on the flat or uphill or even downhill; interval sprints on downhill slopes improve a skier's tempo and balance. Uphill sprints will tax the muscles and the oxygen transport system. Since cross-country ski racing involves so much uphill skiing, a great deal of interval training should be done on hills and hilly loops.

TYPES OF INTERVAL WORKOUTS. Running or bounding uphill with poles is a favorite ski-training interval workout. Although the technique is not quite the same as for hill running on roller skis, the benefits to the oxygen transport system and to the stomach, back, and leg muscles are tremendous. Enough similarities remain to make it quite a specific exercise.

Ski-walking uphill, very fast, is also a good interval workout, as are uphill intervals on bikes and roller skis. Long biking intervals of seven to ten minutes can be done on a good uphill section. A series of forty-five- to sixty-second double-pole intervals on a gradual uphill slope is a terrific workout on roller skis. Running is also good interval training.

Snow-skiing intervals improve tempo and pace as well as Max VO_2. A great variety—long, short, flat, and hilly—is appropriate. For a week or two before major competitions, it is a good rule to keep your heart rate five to fifteen beats below your maximum.

Planning a Lifetime Training Program

The training of young American skiers has perhaps suffered from an inability to see goals as long-term objectives and to exercise patience in achieving them. Programs have been planned to bring skiers to their peak too soon.

The Finnish Ski Association has produced a reasonable plan for skier development in which a skier's career is divided into a number of periods with clearly established goals. If you're a young skier, or the parent or coach of young skiers, you can certainly adapt some of the Finnish objectives to your purposes. And they're probably applicable to serious recreational skiers as well as to developing world-class competitors.

The Finnish scheme divides skiers' ages as follows:

1. 0–10 years   Children with family and friends
2. 11–15 years   The period for learning technique
3. 16–18 years   The serious training years
4. 19–30 years   Competition
5. 31 years and up The years of skiing for oneself

The objectives for children under ten are to build positive experiences by learning to ski together with family and friends, and to create an interest in skiing events. At this earliest age there should be no training, no systematic instruction, and no compulsory participation.

The age for learning technique ranges from eleven to fifteen. Children in this age group who show interest and ability should be encouraged to maintain good health and nutritional habits; to develop their muscles in proportion; to perfect their skiing technique; and to begin training for aerobic capacity. The way to motivate young competitors for the rigorous training that lies ahead is to instruct them in natural methods and freely share information about exercise and training.

For sixteen- to eighteen-year-olds, training should develop aerobic capacity, prepare the body to tolerate hard training, begin developing anaerobic capacity, and promote discipline and character. At this age they usually want to receive comprehensive information about a skier's lifetime program of competition and training.

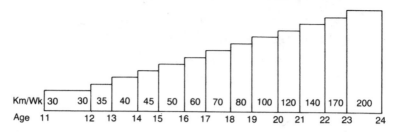

Km/Wk	30		30	35	40	45	50	60	70	80	100	120	140	170	200
Age	11		12	13	14	15	16	17	18	19	20	21	22	23	24

figure 7 (see chapter 3, page 34)

As skiers reach the age range for competition, nineteen to thirty, the objectives change. Now the goals are top performance, consistent results, and total dedication to training. Figure 7 gives rough figures for weekly training distances throughout the year at various ages. The training year, of course, breaks down into the dry-land months of jogging, hiking, biking, and roller-skiing; the preparation for snow; the hard skiing months; and the transition back to dry land.

Around the early thirties, the Finns suggest, is the age for "cooling off." But even after a skier's peak has passed, it's important to maintain good physical condition, to encourage young athletes, and in general to become a public relations advocate for cross-country skiing.

Short-Term Planning. Developing athletes may want to plot out a fairly complete yearly plan. Following are some guidelines for short-term planning that can help you create a comprehensive picture of your development as a skier, whether you are in a team situation, with a coach who will assume some of the responsibility for your training, or generating a training program strictly for your own benefit.

The first step is to summarize your past four years of training activity. See Four-Year Training Summary.

Four-Year Training Summary

NAME: _____

	19___					19___					19___					19___				
	KMS	HRS	RATE	%	AVG. VWL	KMS	HRS	RATE	%	AVG. VWL	KMS	HRS	RATE	%	AVG. VWL	KMS	HRS	RATE	%	AVG. VWL
ENDURANCE TRAINING																				
RUNNING																				
ROLLER-SKIING																				
HIKING																				
BIKING																				
SKIING																				
RACING																				
INTERVALS																				
STRENGTH																				
TOTALS																				

The next step is to establish your base level, determine areas that most need improvement, and make a plan for progress. Some kind of testing will be helpful here. Tests can be simple or incredibly complex, and every coach or team has a different set of favorite measurements with which to compare athletic performance.

Here is a list of tests for specific functions related to cross-country skiing. For each testing area, the following test is a simple one that can be done without special equipment:

Cross-Country Ski Tests
compiled by Dr. Art Dickinson
Colorado University Sportsmedicine Laboratory

Cardiovascular Endurance (Maximum VO_2, Anaerobic Threshold, Lactate Levels)

1. Oxygen consumption levels and related tests on motor-driven treadmill
2. Bicycle ergometer or treadmill *estimate* of endurance capacity using heart rate/work load
3. Twelve-minute run or 1½-mile run plus annual timed speed hike

Muscular Strength (Leg)

1. Isokinetic hydraulic testing apparatus (Cybex machine) —leg extension, hip extension
2. Aircraft cable tensiometer test of leg extension at knee
3. One repetition maximum weight for half squat

Arm-Shoulder Extension

1. Shoulder extension on Cybex machine
2. Aircraft cable tensiometer test of shoulder extension
3. One repetition maximum bench press

Leg Muscle Endurance

1. Cybex (isokinetic hydraulic) measure of strength decrement
2. Strength loss measured by cable tensiometer after one minute of one-legged knee bends (maximum effort)
3. Number of squat jumps in thirty-second period

Arm Muscle Endurance

1. Cybex (isokinetic hydraulic) measure of strength decrement
2. Strength decrement after one-minute arm dips of 45 percent
3. Number of dips in thirty seconds

Body Composition (Percentage Fat)

1. Underwater weighing
2. Skinfold calipers and equation of Pascale (men) or Sloan (women)
3. Abdominal circumference and body-weight equation of Wilmore-Beneke

Power

1. Cybex measures
2. Stair run timed to .001 of a second and vertical jump in foot-pounds of force
3. Standing broad jump for distance and vertical jump in inches

---

The third step is to plan improvement. The following chart will be useful in prospective planning. Please bear in mind that a 20 percent increase or improvement is probably the maximum in any area, and in many cases much less than 20 percent is desirable.

Yearly Plan

Goals	April–July	August–October	November–December	January–March	Total Overall
Total Distance					
Running					
Roller-Skiing					
Hiking					
Biking					
Skiing					
% Endurance Hrs					
% Interval Hrs					
% Strength Hrs					
% Race Hrs					
Total Hours					

Improvement Goals:
April–July:
August–October:
November–December:
Competition Period:
Overall Goals:

The last step is adjustment of the program. No plan is foolproof; all must be reevaluated constantly. Make it a point to adjust your program every six weeks, whether you're working with a coach or alone. Almost everyone begins with unrealistic expectations of performance. Don't be discouraged if you fall short of the goals you have set for yourself. Be realistic; set them lower.

Training Logs. The training log is an indispensable part of program planning. Future programs must be based on past experiences, and the training log is an athlete's record of both subjective and objective experience. A well-kept log will include information about (1) signs and feelings of approaching illness, (2) signs and feelings of approaching peaks, (3) the sequence of workouts that lead up to either overtraining or undertraining, (4) the effect of injuries on training, (5) the effectiveness of workout sequences in accomplishing objectives, and (6) the effect of outside forces—schoolwork, emotional-family problems, world events, weather—on training.

Keeping a log is fun. Training can be an adventure in self-awareness. When you have kept a log faithfully for a season or more, you'll be able to look back at high points, low points, and everything in between to discover your personal strengths and weaknesses and to understand yourself better.

4.
neuromuscular training for strength and power

MUSCULAR STRENGTH is the basis of all human movement. For skiers, strength is necessary not only to move the body forward but also to change direction quickly and maintain balance. Also, increasing strength is the only demonstrated method of increasing agility significantly. Agility test scores have improved as much as 50 percent as strength is improved.

Strength is the measure of force produced when thousands of muscle fibers shorten in unison, exerting a pull on a tendon that connects the fibers to a bone. The amount of force produced depends on the number of fibers, in groups of 15 to 1,500, that are stimulated by the motor neurons of the nervous system to contract. These groups of muscle fibers, called *motor units*, always shorten to their maximum capability when stimulated, so the amount of force produced depends on how many motor units contract. When we first try to perform a movement like the leg drive and glide of cross-country skiing, many motor units contract that are not necessary to the motion. As we improve, many of these wasteful muscular contractions are eliminated. And as we perform the movements more efficiently, otherwise wasted energy is conserved. Over a distance of several kilometers, this difference is striking.

If a skier isn't strong enough to perform a movement efficiently, supplementary muscular force will be recruited from areas in a less favorable line of pull. As groups of muscles are depleted of their stored fuel, they become fatigued and their contractile force diminishes. Other muscles must compensate in order to keep up the pace of forward movement. When a skier lacks strength or is fatigued, form deteriorates, efficiency drops, and energy expenditure increases dramatically, leading to deeper fatigue and threatening exhaustion.

Strength Training. Strength isn't simply the ability to generate a single maximum effort. It is a continuum, with a single maximum effort at one end and the ability to repeat submaximal efforts with undiminished force at the other. The repetitive capacity is sometimes called endurance, but it is a mistake for cross-country skiers to regard the two ends as separate; we need to develop both ends of the continuum.

If a muscle is forced to contract against great resistance, with only a few repetitions, then the principal change in the muscle tissue will be an increase in the contractile protein of the cells, called the *actin* and *myosin* filaments.

With lighter resistance and many repetitions, the predominant change will be an increase in the energy-producing proteins of the cell—oxidative enzymes, mitochondria, and myoglobin. Cross-country skiers have intermittent needs for maximum-strength contractions but a constant need for submaximal muscular contractions with no deterioration in performance. Therefore, the second type of strength training is more appropriate.

Muscular *power* is defined as work done per unit of time. A weight lifter may have great strength, but, for example, inadequate power to be a shot-putter. In spite of his great strength, he doesn't have the speed of movement to accelerate the resistance of a 16-pound shot.

Power can also be defined as "explosion." Because skiers need endurance, and skeletal muscles contribute as much to endurance as the cardiovascular system does, most cross-country skiers don't have great muscle power. Muscle biopsies of cross-country skiers confirm the predominance of high-endurance capacity, slow-twitch red fibers with low contractile speed.

The strength-training program for a cross-country skier should consist primarily of endurance-building exercises that will increase contractile force to some extent, and secondarily of exercises for high force development.

Strength is a secondary sex characteristic and is dependent on blood testosterone levels. That is why the average woman has only 65 to 70 percent of the muscle strength of the average man. Women can improve their strength, however, at the same rate as men with a resistance-exercise program. Male-female strength differences are greater in the arms than in the legs. Because the arms are so important in cross-country skiing, women should pay particular attention to resistance exercises for the arms, shoulders, chest, and upper back.

Strength is gained rapidly in the first three weeks of a training program, partly because of nervous-system training; the athlete learns how it feels to exert a near-maximum contraction. After six weeks, the rate of improvement slows.

When a strength-training program is stopped, strength is lost much more slowly than it was gained. Once a desired level of strength has been achieved, it can usually be maintained by once- or twice-a-week workouts. Start your strength-building program in late spring. It will involve three or four sessions weekly for twelve to sixteen weeks, and strength-maintenance programs after that.

The Exercise Program. The exercise program has three objectives:

1. To develop enough muscular strength to challenge terrain with adequate power and endurance;
2. To maintain desired tempo without fatigue that would cause technique to deteriorate and energy cost to increase;
3. To summon the power necessary to shift body mass or change direction instantly in order to maintain balance, run a course efficiently, or protect against injury.

The following general principles should be kept in mind when you plan your strength-training program:

- Your strength-training program should be an efficient time investment. Don't work on muscle groups that aren't directly involved in cross-country skiing.

- Your training program should be specific. Your resistance exercises should duplicate as closely as possible the joint angles and planes of movement used in cross-country skiing.
- Strength requirements differ among skiers. More powerful skiers can do less resistance exercise. Less powerful skiers will find that their capacity to increase muscular strength is high; training will yield gratifying results.
- The changes aren't as dramatically visible as changes in strength, but your resistance-exercise program will increase the density and tensile strength of your ligaments and tendons. The main reason for strengthening these connective tissues is to protect you against injury or reinjury.
- Stretching, both before and after resistance exercise, is worth the ten or fifteen minutes it takes. But if you can't do both, stretching *after* resistance exercise is more important for maintaining flexibility.

Types of Resistance Exercise. Resistance exercise is any type of overload training that causes adaptive changes in the quality of muscular contraction. Hill striding, bounding, running, and high-gear cycling are all types of resistance exercise, although athletes generally use them as interval workouts for general endurance or power (see Chapter 3); but power—work done per unit of time—is one demonstration of strength.

Activities such as one-legged or two-legged repeat jumps, parallel-bar dips, pack hiking, pack striding, or pack knee-dips can also be resistance exercise; so can one leg or arm resisting the movement of the other, or one person resisting another.

ISOMETRIC EXERCISE. Isometric (static) exercise is muscular contraction against a resistance greater than the muscle's maximum strength. In isometrics, no joint movement occurs. This method generates maximum muscular force. Although it is often used for post-injury rehabilitation, static exercise has no particular usefulness in a cross-country exercise program because it doesn't increase muscular endurance or muscle strength throughout the range of motion.

ISOTONIC EXERCISE. Isotonic (dynamic) exercise is muscular contraction that is stronger than the resistance. Isotonics involves joint movement, either through muscle shortening, called *concentric contraction,* or through controlled lengthening of the muscle, called *eccentric contraction.*

A concentric contraction is the action of the biceps flexing the elbow to help lift the body upward on a chinning bar. The same biceps working to return the body slowly to its starting position gives an example of a lengthening or eccentric contraction.

Most resistance exercises are isotonic. The only disadvantages of these exercises is that the maximum resistance is limited to the weakest angle of the joint moving through its range of motion. Therefore, strengthening won't be efficient in some parts of the movement where the muscle is capable of working against a heavier load.

Lengthening contractions require less than half the energy needed for shortening contractions.

ISOKINETIC EXERCISE. Isokinetic exercise is muscular contraction against a resistance that varies with the magnitude of force available at different joint angles. *Accommodating resistance* might be a better term for it. As the muscle moves the joint through its range of motion, the resistance will increase or decrease with the sum of the forces able to act at each radian of movement.

The best isokinetic exercise is obtained from commercial systems. Research indicates that isokinetic resistance exercise is the most effective method of strength training, but the equipment is not generally available. Also, the limited positions for exercises appropriate for skiers seriously restrict the value of isokinetic resistance-exercise programs —other than partner-resistance activities, like wrestling.

Major Muscles. Some muscle groups, such as the shoulder and arm extensors, work importantly over long periods, while others, such as the outward rotators of the leg, con-

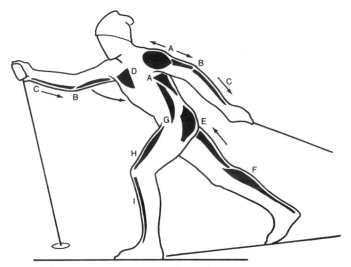

figure 1 Muscle involvement in diagonal stride: A. Shoulder extension; B. Elbow extension; C. Wrist adduction; D. Scapula adduction and rotation; E. Hip extension; F. Ankle plantar flexion (extension); G. Hip flexion; H. Knee extension; I. Ankle dorsiflexion.

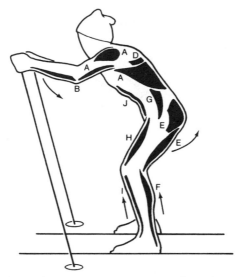

figure 2 Muscle involvement in double-poling: A. Shoulder extension; B. Elbow and wrist stabilization; D. Scapula down rotation and adduction; E. Hip extension; F. Ankle plantar flexion; G. Trunk flexion (hip flexion); H. Leg extension at knee; I. Ankle dorsiflexion; J. Trunk flexion (abdominal muscles).

tribute short bursts of powerful contractions, as in herringboning.

The following classification of the body's major muscle groups lists their importance for cross-country skiing, both primarily and secondarily. A fourth category of muscles is listed because it can help to minimize the effects of injury. (Figures 1–5)

Muscles of the Trunk
- Abdominals—used strongly in double-poling. Also provide a stable base, with the back extensors and the trunk rotators, for the leg muscles in every position.
- Back extensors—control the degree of tuck and work with other trunk muscles.
- Trunk rotators.

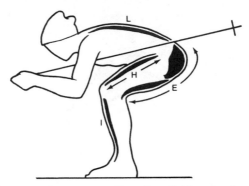

figure 3 Muscle involvement — tuck position: E. Hip extension; I. Ankle dorsiflexion; L. Back extension, knee extension. (All important in controlling tuck angles.)

Shoulder-Arm Muscles

- Upper arm and shoulder extensors (among others, the posterior deltoid, triceps, and latissimus dorsi) and scapula adductors—provide the force for both single- and double-poling.
- Elbow extensors (triceps and anconeus) and wrist adductors—maintain a semirigid joint so the upper arm and shoulder drive can be transmitted to the pole without loss of force. These muscles can become sore from roller-ski poling on road surfaces.

Hip and Leg Muscles.

- Hip extensors (among others, the gluteus maximus and hamstring muscles)—provide much of the forward power thrust, support part of the body weight during the glide phase, and help to regulate the tuck position on downhills.
- Hip flexors—also used in thrust, but don't have to exert as much force as the hip extensors.
- Knee extensors (quadriceps group)—must work

strongly with hip extensors for leg drive and help to support body weight during glide. Also, with the hip extensors, control the degree of tuck on the downhill.

- Angle flexors—these muscles, on the front side of the lower leg, are important as stabilizers in properly transferring force and body weight to the ski.
- Ankle extensors—muscles at the rear of the lower leg; assist in transfer of force or body weight and add a "flip" of final force to the backward thrust of the ski on snow.
- Outward rotators—most important for herringboning.

The hip extensors, knee extensors, and shoulder-arm extensors are the muscles that determine a skier's quality of performance. Along with the stabilizing function of the

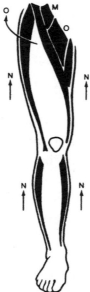

figure 4 Rotators and lateral stabilizers of leg — important in tuck and uphill: M. Outward rotation of leg at thigh; N. Lateral stabilization at knee and ankle; O. Abduct legion.

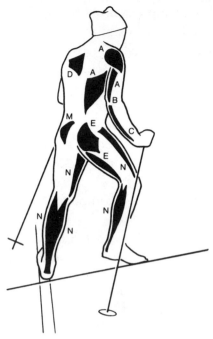

figure 5 Muscle involvement — herringbone: A. and D. Shoulder extension; B. and C. Elbow and wrist stabilization; E. Hip extension; M. Outward rotation of leg at thigh; N. and F. Lateral stabilization at knee and ankle.

trunk muscles and foot flexor muscles, a cross-country ski racer's success will be determined by the contractile force and endurance capability of these muscles.

Injury Minimization. Muscles that play a part in minimizing injury include those of the shoulder, knee, and elbow joints.

At the *shoulder joint,* developing the strength of the muscles that bring the arm in to the body, rotate the lower arm across the body, and lift the arm outward and forward will help to prevent serious shoulder problems in falls.

At the *knee joint,* the quadriceps, hamstrings, and inward and outward rotators all help to stabilize the knee joint against injury.

At the *elbow joint,* the muscles that flex and extend the wrist help to transmit force from the shoulder and arm to the pole and are vulnerable to overuse injury.

Designing a Program. No single exercise program will meet every athlete's needs. However, the following table should allow the enthusiastic skier to design her or his own efficient program of neuromuscular activities for strength and power.

Weight workouts generally last from forty-five to ninety minutes and involve two or three sets of eight to twelve well-chosen exercises. In the preceding table, Grade I movements are those that are absolutely necessary to a cross-country resistance-exercise program, Grade II movements are those that should be in the program if time and equipment permit, and Grade III movements are exercises that contribute to prevention or minimization of injury.

Grade I Movements

MOVEMENT	MAJOR MUSCLES	TYPE OF RESISTANCE EXERCISE*
Hip extension	Gluteus maximus Hamstrings	HE, HF →
Knee extension	Quadriceps	HE, HF

Combined hip and knee extension ------------------------------------

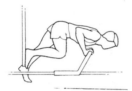
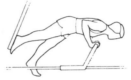

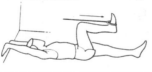

Shoulder-arm extension and scapula adduction	Posterior deltoid, triceps, latissimus dorsi, trapeziums, rhomboids	HE, HF

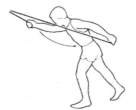

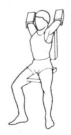

* HE—HIGH ENDURANCE
HF—HIGH FORCE

1. Nautilus gear, leg and back

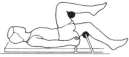

2. Free weights, half squats

1. Lumex "Orthotron"
2. Universal leg extension table
3. Nautilus leg exercise machine

1. Universal hip and knee press station, one leg at a time
2. Free weights, jumping or walking squats
3. Hiking, roller-skiing, uphill
4. Nautilus compound leg machine (also use backward)
5. Hill bounding; wall squats with backpack; one-legged jump squats
6. Atlas (Exergenie) resistance to running motion
7. Mini-gym "leaper"

1. Atlas (Exergenie)
2. Roller board, kneeling position
3. Universal lateral pull machine
4. Nautilus combination pullover torso

(continued)

Grade I Movements

MOVEMENT	MAJOR MUSCLES	TYPE OF RESISTANCE EXERCISE*
Elbow extension and wrist adduction	Triceps, anconeus, flexors, and extensors on ulnar side of wrist	HE, HF
Ankle dorsiflexion	Anterior tibial muscle, long extensor muscles of toes	HE
Hip flexion, trunk or pelvis	Rectus abdominis, internal and external oblique muscles of abdomen 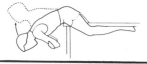	HE, HF

Grade II Movements

MOVEMENT	MAJOR MUSCLES	TYPE OF RESISTANCE EXERCISE*
Hip flexion, thigh on pelvis	Pectineal muscle, iliopsoas, straight muscle of thigh 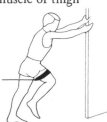	HE 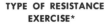

* HE—HIGH ENDURANCE
HF—HIGH FORCE

1. Atlas (Exergenie)
2. Roller board
3. Universal lateral pull
4. Wood chopping
5. Free weights, pullover, bench press

---

1. Atlas (Exergenie)
2. Self-resistance—resist one foot with the other
3. Ankle flexions against mattress
4. Hiking on uneven terrain

---

1. "Good mornings" or sit-ups with Atlas (Exergenie)
2. Bent-knee sit-ups with barbell plate
3. Universal slant board
4. Alternate knee-to-elbow sit-ups from supine position

EXERCISE

1. Atlas (Exergenie), using strap at midthigh
2. High knee lifts, with barbell plate on thigh
3. Bicycle sprints uphill, using toe clips

(continued)

Grade II Movements

MOVEMENT	MAJOR MUSCLES	TYPE OF RESISTANCE EXERCISE*
Back extension	Erector spinae	HE →
Hip outward rotation	6 deep outward rotators, gluteus maximus, biceps femoris	HF
Upper- and lower-leg lateral stabilizers	Adductor group, gluteus medius and minimum, tensor fasciae latae, peroneals, posterior tibial muscle, long flexors of the toes	HF
Ankle extension, plantar flexion	Gastrocnemius, soleus, posterior tibial	HE

* HE—HIGH ENDURANCE
HF—HIGH FORCE

1. Atlas (Exergenie)
2. Free weights, extension "good mornings," dead lift, military press
3. Bench-lying extensions with barbell plate

---

1. Atlas (Exergenie)
2. Free weights, extension "good mornings," dead lift, military press
3. Bench-lying extensions with barbell plate

---

1. Atlas (Exergenie) in sitting position with strap immediately below knee
2. Free weights, hip rotations in standing position, barbell resting on shoulders
3. Free weights, barbell squats with knees outward

---

1. Free weights, toe raises
2. Universal—toe raises

(continued)

Grade II Movements

MOVEMENT	MAJOR MUSCLES	TYPE OF RESISTANCE EXERCISE*
Trunk rotation	External and internal oblique abdominals, transverse and straight abdominals	HF

Grade III Movements

MOVEMENT	MAJOR MUSCLES	TYPE OF RESISTANCE EXERCISE*
Inward rotation and adduction of shoulder	Subscapular, teres major, rotator cuff	HF $\longrightarrow$
Abduction and flexion of shoulder	Deltoid, rotator cuff	HF
Knee extension	Quadriceps	HF
Knee flexion	Hamstrings	HF
Knee inward and outward rotation	Great muscles of leg, sartorius, tensor muscles of the fascia, hamstrings	HF

* HE—HIGH ENDURANCE
HF—HIGH FORCE

1. Free weights, trunk rotation with weight on shoulders
2. Free weights, trunk lateral bends with weight on shoulders
3. Atlas (Exergenie), pull across chest, using trunk muscles

---

1. Atlas (Exergenie)
2. Universal or Marcy pulley weight cable

---

1. Free weights, lateral raises (dumbbells), forward raises (dumbbells), military press, upright rows, bench press
2. Atlas (Exergenie)

See Grade I Movements

---

1. Universal or Marcy leg curl machine
2. Nautilus leg curl machine
3. Resist one leg with the other

---

1. Atlas (Exergenie) with strap immediately below knee
2. Partner or individual resistance

5.
training for coordination, balance, agility, flexibility, and relaxation

BALANCE, coordination, agility, and flexibility are important enough to cross-country skiing performance that attention must be specifically paid to them in any training program. However, since training for these skills isn't as strenuous as cardiovascular and strength-training workouts, it can usually be incorporated into the more exhausting activities.

Coordination, Balance and Agility

Roller-skiing. Technically, correct roller-skiing is the most specific dry-land training for skiers and will result in the best muscle-memory carryover to snow skiing. It is basic to development of balance and coordination.

Balance Beam. A good balance exercise for skiers uses a series of two-by-fours or two-by-sixes, turned on edge and bolted at each end to two posts. Place them at various heights and angles and have fun. Walking and doing exercise routines on these beams, while not specific to skiing, make for good training for overall balance and coordination.

Woods Running. Running in fairly open forest has long been a favorite exercise for cross-country skiers. The Swedes call it *fartlek,* or speed play. It can be part of a natural interval workout. Running up and down hills, in and out of trees, is good for balance, coordination, and agility, and it trains skiers to watch for stumps, holes, and other hazards.

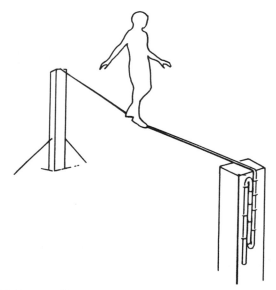

figure 1 Tightrope walking can be fun and good for balance. A tightrope walk is easy to build in the back yard. Stretch a ¾" to 1" rope between two trees or sunken 4" x 6" posts. The rope should be about 5 feet off the ground at the ends and should be prestretched. A winch or come-along may be needed to tighten the rope, which should be stretched as tightly as possible between the two trees or posts.

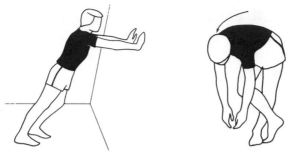

figure 2   Lean against wall with arms and forearms fully extended and feet flat on the floor. The calves of the legs are fully extended alternately. Hold each stretch for 30 seconds.

figure 3   Posterior tissue stretch. Cross one leg over the other and rest toes of crossed leg at outer edge of other foot. This will stretch only one leg at a time. Alternate legs.

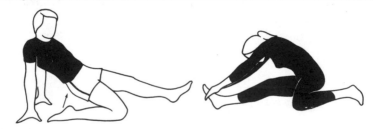

figure 4-a   Thigh stretches. Back-lying position to start, with one leg extended. Bent-knee leg has toes extended to rear. Lift hips upward to stretch thigh of bent leg. Alternate legs.

figure 4-b   Traditional "hurdler's stretch." Forward leg does *not* have to be locked at knee joint.

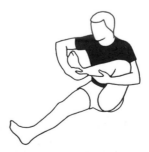

figure 5   Posterior and leg-adductor tissue stretch. Gently pull leg into body and rotate leg inward with both arms.

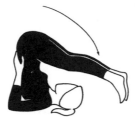

figure 6 Hip stretch. Support low-back area with both hands.

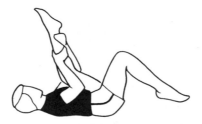

figure 7 Low-back and posterior tissue stretch. Use both arms to pull straightened leg gently toward chest. Let opposite leg hang in bent position.

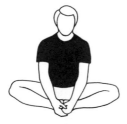 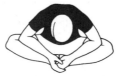

figure 8 Lower-back, groin, posterior tissue stretch. Put the soles of the feet together and grab toes. Slowly pull yourself down. Hold position for 20-30 seconds.

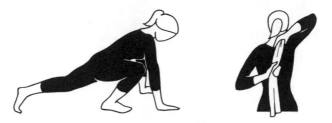

figure 9 Hip and thigh stretch. Let forward knee rotate outward until stretch is felt on inner side of thigh (adductor muscles).

figure 10 Back and shoulder stretch. Grasp towel, ski pole, etc., and use alternate arms to exert gentle stretch in several joint angles.

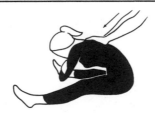

figure 11 Full stretch. The person being stretched opens the legs as far as possible, keeping knees straight and heels on floor. The person giving the stretch should apply slow, even pressure with the hands to the middle portion of the back of the person being stretched. This pressure should be slow and directly forward, until the "stretchee" feels tension in the groin area. Hold this position for 20-30 seconds.

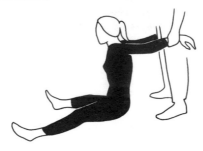

Next, in the same seated position, the stretcher grabs both the stretchee's arms at the wrist and gently pulls the arms back and slightly up until the stretchee feels the muscles in the chest being stretched. Hold this position for 20-30 seconds.

Soccer, Tennis, and Other Sports. Many coaches have discouraged ski racers from playing soccer because of the game's potential for injury. But soccer played properly is excellent training for balance and eye-foot coordination. It should be played on a smooth, level, prepared field. Players shouldn't wear soccer shoes but ski boots. This will prevent injuries and force players to balance better over their feet.

Many skiers play tennis, including most members of the U.S. Cross-Country Team. The balance, coordination, and lateral movements involved make it an excellent change of pace for ski racers. Any sport, in fact, that stresses balance and is safe is good training for cross-country skiers.

Flexibility

An athlete must be concerned with both the range of motion about a joint and the opposition or resistance of the joint to motion. Good ski technique isn't possible without flexibility. This is one of the most neglected areas in a typical cross-country training program.

The best flexibility exercises are the so-called stretching exercises which are illustrated on the preceding pages. They should be performed passively; that is, without bobbing or forcing. Stretch unhurriedly and hold the final, fully elongated position for up to forty-five seconds. This takes less energy, provides less risk of injury during warm-up, and relieves soreness better.

The passive stretching program should be done three to six times per week for fifteen to thirty minutes each time. You'll notice improvement in a couple of weeks, as you're able to hold positions longer and do the exercises more often. If one muscle group is particularly stiff, spend more time on stretches for that group.

Stretches should bring the body to the point of tension but not pain. Hold each position for fifteen to forty-five seconds, then repeat. Concentrate on the stretch.

Heel-cord and lower-leg stretch. Stand 3 feet from a flat wall; place palms flat against wall. Keeping heels flat on floor, stretch in position A, with one knee bent. Follow with position B, straightening that knee and bending the opposite one.

Alternate legs.

Relaxation

Relaxation is one of the most overlooked aspects of training. Like other skills, it takes practice and concentration: the body must learn how to relax.

Ability to relax mentally from the stress of training, competition, and travel results in more rested athletes who are better able to compete at their optimum level. Ability to relax physically will enable you to move more economically and skillfully.

The following routine is described as though a coach were leading a small team of ski racers through it, but it is adaptable to your private use, either with or without a partner. This routine should be done once a week.

The environment in which the relaxation routine is to be performed is important. The room should be dark, warm, and quiet, with fresh air. You should lie on a carpet or a blanket. Soft music often aids in relaxation.

Begin by lying on your back. If you're doing this with a leader or a partner, the leader should suggest that you concentrate on relaxing and on each major muscle group, tendon, joint, organ, and painful area of the body, beginning with the toes and working up to the head. If you're doing this alone, it will help you to write out a script and memorize it.

Focus only on the area being examined and relaxed. No other thoughts should enter your mind. The relaxation routine should take between forty-five minutes and an hour. If you fall asleep during it, that means you're not getting enough rest. Do it again when you're fully rested. Relaxation is such an important part of your training that you should stay awake for it.

THE RIGHT LEG. Relax each individual toe. Relax the arch of the foot, which is tense after a day of supporting the body mass. Mentally take apart your heel and examine all its parts. Mentally examine the parts of your foot that may hurt after a day of skiing. Focus on your inside and outside calf muscles, and relax them. Mentally take apart your knee joint and polish the knee cap. Focus on relaxing the muscles along the inside of your thigh, stretching from the kneecap to the crotch. Focus on relaxing the quadriceps muscle along the top of your thigh, from kneecap to hip. Focus on the muscle along the outside of your thigh, from kneecap to hip. Focus on the hamstring muscles that stretch from the back of the knee to the buttocks.

THE LEFT LEG. Follow the same sequence.

ABDOMINAL MUSCLES. Divide the abdominal muscles into three bands that encircle the trunk. Focus on relaxing each band separately.

BACK AND VERTEBRAE. Visualize the two large muscles that run along each side of the vertebrae. These muscles support the vertebrae, which are stacked on top of one another like china plates. The two muscles run from the coccyx, or tailbone, all the way to the neck. Concentrate on relaxing each of the two muscle groups separately. Focus on each vertebra from the coccyx to the base of the skull.

NECK.

RIBS. Spend time focusing on each rib, moving up to the collarbone.

LUNGS.

HEART.

RIGHT SHOULDER JOINT. Take the joint apart and examine each part. Focus on the triceps and biceps muscles, from shoulder joint to elbow. Focus on the elbow joint. Take it apart and examine the parts. Focus on the muscles of the forearm. Focus on the wrist and relax it. Examine each individual finger.

LEFT SHOULDER JOINT. Follow the same sequence.

THROAT.

JAW.

TONGUE.

LIPS.

NOSE.

LEFT EYE, RIGHT EYE. Mentally remove each eye and examine it separately.

LEFT EYELID, RIGHT EYELID. Relax each one separately.

FOREHEAD. The forehead is the source of much tension. Concentrate on relaxing it so that the wrinkles disappear.

LEFT EAR, RIGHT EAR. Examine each ear separately, inside and out.

HEAD. Focus on the skull and scalp, moving from back to front. Go inside the skull and shut down the computer. Eliminate all anxieties and worries. Visualize a peaceful scene where you feel relaxed and secure, such as by a lake or on a beach.

Remain in this relaxed state for about five minutes. You may find it useful to make a tape cassette of this relaxation routine so that you can play it and not have to remember the sequence of elements.

An Alternate Method. Here is another, similar routine. The primary focus of this routine is to learn how it feels to have your muscles first truly tense and then truly relaxed. At each step you are asked first to tense up a muscle group and then to relax it, paying close attention to how the muscles feel. Tense up each muscle group for only as long as you need to learn how it feels—about five seconds. Relax the muscle group for about the same amount of time.

These times are approximate. Don't let yourself be distracted by paying too much attention to counting or timing. Just tense up the muscles until you can really feel the tension, and then relax them.

The routine follows a systematic pattern: dominant hand, other hand; right biceps, left biceps; forehead, eyes, facial area; chest, abdomen; legs; and feet. When you begin, repeat twice for each group before going to the next group. Later, when you're familiar with the routine, you can omit first the repetition and then the tension; you'll be able simply to relax each muscle group in turn.

After relaxing each muscle group, permit it to remain relaxed. The first time you do this relaxation routine, either have someone read the instructions aloud for you or put them on a tape cassette. The instructions should be read in a normal voice. It will help to pace the exercise if the reader —your partner or yourself when you make the tape—does the routine while speaking. The aim of the exercise is to tense the muscle group long enough for its effect to be noticeable, but not long enough so that it is painful or will lead to cramps or fatigue.

Some muscle groups, like those around the eyes, the jaw, and the feet, should be tensed for only about three seconds, to avoid pain or cramping.

Choose a time of day when you will not be disturbed. Many athletes practice just before going to bed; they find the relaxation achieved helps them to fall asleep. Get into a comfortable position, preferably that of lying on your back. Use a small pillow for your head if you wish.

Close your eyes so as not to be distracted by your surroundings. Now, tense your dominant hand into a fist . . . as tight as you can get it . . . so that you can feel the tension . . . really tight, the tighter the better, you can really feel the tension . . . Now relax the hand, letting the tension remove itself . . . feeling the muscles become loose . . . Notice the contrast between the tension of moments before and the relaxation, the absence of tension . . . Allow the fingers to relax, and then the entire dominant hand. (Repeat.)

Now we'll leave the dominant hand and focus on the other hand. Tense your other hand by making it into a fist . . . very tight . . . and again, notice how the tension feels . . . Focus on the tense muscles . . . All right, now relax the hand . . . and notice the contrast between the tension of a moment ago and the relaxation . . . Continue to be aware of the relaxation of the muscles . . . in the fingers . . . and throughout the entire hand. (Repeat.)

We'll leave the hands and fingers relaxed and now move to the arms, the biceps . . . In order to tense the biceps, you'll have to bend the arm at the elbow, tightening your biceps muscle by moving your hand toward your shoulder. Let's start with the right arm.

Bend your right arm at the elbow so that your hand moves toward your shoulder . . . tight . . . keep tightening up the biceps as hard as you can . . . focus your attention on the muscle tension . . . really notice how that feels . . . Now relax . . . let the arm and hand drop back down . . . and notice the relaxation, the absence of tension . . . Feel the relaxation as it takes over the upper arm . . . Notice the feeling of relaxation in the lower arm, in the hand and fingers. (Repeat.)

Now we'll leave the right arm relaxed and move to the left arm. Tense up the left arm by bending it at the elbow . . . really tense, as tense as you can get it . . . and focus your attention on the feelings of tension . . . Now relax, let your arm drop back down . . . Notice the difference in feeling between the tension and the relaxation . . . permit the relaxation to take over the entire left arm . . . the upper arm . . . the forearm . . . the hands . . . and the fingers. (Repeat.)

We'll leave the hands and arms comfortably relaxed and move on to the forehead. In order to tense up the forehead, you must frown.

All right, I want you to tense your forehead by frowning

. . . *Wrinkle up the forehead area . . . very tight . . . and notice how the tension feels . . . Now relax . . . Let the wrinkles smooth themselves out . . . Allow the relaxation to proceed on its own . . . making the forehead as smooth and tension-free as though you were passing your hand over a sheet to smooth it out. (Repeat.)*

We'll leave the forehead relaxed . . . and move on to the eyes . . . What I want you to do is to close your eyes tighter than they are . . . tighter . . . feeling the tension (use less time for tension here, to avoid afterimages) . . . Now relax . . . keeping the eyes comfortably closed . . . Notice the contrast between tension and relaxation. (Repeat.)

Notice the relaxation in the right hand and fingers . . . and the feeling of relaxation in the forearm and upper arm . . . Notice the relaxation in the left hand and fingers . . . in the forearm and upper arm . . . Let the relaxation take over and include the forehead . . . smooth and without tension.. . . the eyes . . . the facial area . . . and the lips and jaw.

We'll now proceed to help the relaxation across the chest. I want you to tense up the chest muscles by taking a deep breath and holding it for a moment . . . Notice the tension . . . Now exhale slowly, breathe normally again . . . and notice the chest muscles as they become more and more relaxed. (Repeat.)

Now we'll move on to the abdomen . . . I want you to tense up your abdominal muscles right now . . . very tight . . . Pay attention to the tension . . . Now relax . . . Let the feeling of relaxation take over . . . Notice the difference between the feeling of tension a moment ago and the relaxation now. (Repeat.)

On to the legs . . . To tense up your legs and feet, I

want you to point your toes downward until you can feel the muscles of your legs tense up . . . Notice the tension (use tension only for about three seconds, to avoid cramping of the toe or foot muscles) . . . Now relax . . . let the relaxation take over . . . feel the release. (Repeat.)

All right, now simply enjoy the sense of relaxation and comfort across your body . . . Feel loose and relaxed in the hands and fingers . . . comfortable in the forearms and upper arms . . . Notice the relaxed feeling as it includes the forehead . . . the eyes . . . the facial area . . . the lips and jaw . . . Let the relaxation include the chest . . . the abdomen . . . and both legs and both feet.

Now, to further increase the relaxation, I want you to take a deep breath and exhale slowly . . . Use your rhythmical, deep breathing to deepen the relaxation and to permit you to become as relaxed as you want to be . . . Breathe slowly in and out . . . Use your rhythm to achieve whatever level of relaxation you want . . . In future, you may use this deep-breathing technique to initiate or deepen relaxation whenever you want to.

All right, that's fine . . . let your breathing continue normally. In a moment, I'll count backward from 3 to 1 . . . When I get to 1, you'll feel alert and refreshed . . . no aches or pains . . . You can retain the relaxed feeling as long as you wish . . . All right, 3 . . . more and more alert . . . 2 . . . no aches or pains . . . and 1 . . . you can open your eyes . . .

Once you have used the exercise under someone's direction, either that of a skiing partner or your own voice on tape, you can practice relaxation alone by simply tensing and relaxing each muscle group in sequence.

After three or four practice sessions, you can omit the

tension and concentrate on letting each muscle group in sequence become relaxed or limp. With training, you can develop relaxation within five minutes. With much practice, some athletes can initiate relaxation control in one minute. Some athletes are able to use the relaxation technique while sitting on chairs or riding in vehicles, or before competition. Control in relaxing specific muscle groups is possible with repetition.

Repeating the deep-breath technique can help you to initiate relaxation on a quick reflex basis.

Although the relaxation exercise may be used for other forms of training, the directions here are aimed at teaching you how to control your muscle groups to achieve relaxation. As with any other exercise, success with this one requires practice and adherence to the exercise steps. Once a day, five days out of seven, is a normal routine. More frequent use, such as every day, will speed up training.

You will find that the specific training activities outlined in this chapter—exercises for coordination, balance, and agility; stretches for flexibility; and relaxation routines —will have a synergistic effect. That is, doing each one will increase your results from all the others. These refinements of training, combined with your own cross-country training program, will make you a better skier.

6.
nutrition
for
Nordic
skiers

FOR THE cross-country skier, as for most athletes, no part of training except avoidance or physical injury is as important as optimal nutrition. From the food you eat come the material for body development and the fuel for muscular activity—the muscular activity that propels you through thousands of training kilometers as well as through the 5- to 50-kilometer race courses.

Unfortunately, nutrition is a complex and still-developing area of research, with many unknowns and much misinformation, tradition, and faddism. However, enough sound information is presently available to guide skiers in good sports nutrition and to lessen their concern that other athletes may be performing better because of what they are eating.

First, two important facts about sports nutrition should be generally known but are not:

1. Athletes don't belong on a nutritional pedestal. You can't digest tin cans, but if you eat meals well balanced among fats, carbohydrates, and proteins, you won't be far from an ideal sports diet.
2. Below-par sports performance attributable to diet are uncommon. Technique, motivation, quality of training, and systemic illness are much more important variables.

Two principal elements of diet, carbohydrates and fats, serve one primary purpose: they are the fuels, in combination with oxygen, that provide energy for the constant metabolic needs of all body cells, including, of course, the muscle cells. Skeletal muscle cells, as we learned in Chapter 3, are uniquely able to produce energy from carbohydrates for short periods of time, even if adequate oxygen is not present. This anaerobic process is grossly inefficient and produces only 5 percent of the energy possible when sufficient oxygen is present for aerobic metabolism. But during the parts of a ski race that require more energy than the body's aerobic metabolism can supply, the anaerobic process must make up the balance.

The unit of measurement of food energy is the kilocalorie. The average woman ski racer requires from 2800 to 4000 calories daily in hard training; the average man, 4100 to 5300.

Relative amounts of carbohydrates and fat eaten should

depend on the intensity of work. About half the energy necessary for easy skiing will come from fat, whereas in a race, depending on the distance, only 10 to 25 percent of the required energy will come from metabolism of adipose tissue.

Basic Nutrients

Carbohydrates. For anyone, skier or sedentary slob, carbohydrates should predominate in the diet. The normal diet should be from 50 to 55 percent carbohydrate; the ski racer's diet, 55 to 65 percent. We ingest carbohydrates in the form of simple sugars—monosaccharides or disaccharides—or complex sugars—the starches. Both kinds are converted in the body to primary energy fuel: glucose.

Glucose produced and not immediately used can be stored for later use as *glycogen.* About three-fourths of your stored glycogen is within the muscle cells, and the rest is in your liver. However, glycogen storage requires that each gram of glucose must be combined with 2.7 grams of water; therefore, relatively small amounts of glucose—about 2000 calories, or roughly a pound—are stored as glycogen. The rest is converted to a more compact form that needs little accompanying water: *fat.* You probably have between 80,000 and 100,000 calories of potential energy stored as fat in various parts of your body: the thighs, between the shoulder blades, around the lower trunk, and other sites familiar to all.

Carbohydrate is inferior to fat in its storage characteristics and in its energy yield per gram (4.1 calories per gram as against 9.3 calories per gram for fat), but it has two distinct advantages as a fuel for muscular work. First, its breakdown requires less oxygen than that of fat, and therefore it is about 8 percent more efficient in using that vital resource. Second, it produces energy much faster. Additionally, only carbohydrate can produce any energy at all under anaerobic conditions.

During physical activity, the muscles use primarily the carbohydrate stored in the cells, rather than what is circulating in the bloodstream. This means that one limiting factor in cross-country skiing performance will be the amount of carbohydrate stored in muscles. This amount— about 1.5 percent of the total wet weight of the muscle— can be increased to some extent, through training and under some other conditions that will be described later in this chapter.

High-carbohydrate foods include cereals, bread, most vegetables and fruits, and any foods or drinks that are high in sugar. Sugar consumption has its strongly undesirable aspects, but sugar is the most concentrated form of energy. Eating simple sugars in an unrefined form, such as in fruits or honey, is the quickest way for the body to take on usable carbohydrate.

Fats. It is extremely difficult to identify the actual amount of this energy fuel that we eat; even lean meat can be marbled with fat. In digestion, fat breaks down to fatty acids and glycerol and, with adequate oxygen, provides large amounts of energy. One gram, as we saw above, yields 9.3 calories.

Small amounts of fat are stored within the muscle cells, but most of the fat metabolized in skiing will come from the fat repository areas. The average American diet is 35 to 40 percent fat. A more desirable percentage, especially for ski racers, is 15 to 20 percent.

Protein. Tradition in sports dies hard, which is probably the reason for the prevalence of steak and eggs on training tables. However, studies have repeatedly shown that protein contributes nothing as a fuel for muscular activity. To extract enough energy from protein for just a sedentary existence, one would have to consume several pounds of meat at each meal. Most protein eaten in excess of immediate needs is converted to fat.

Nonetheless, protein is basic to human structure and function. Protein is composed of amino acids, of which eight are classified as essential, because we cannot manufacture them within our bodies, and thirteen as nonessential, because we can, if the raw material is available.

Eggs, meat, milk and all dairy products including yogurt and ice cream, fish, and poultry contain all the essential amino acids. At least one essential amino acid is missing from other sources of protein such as legumes, other vegetables, and grains. The athlete who is an ovo-lacto-vegetarian should have few nutritional problems. But vegetarians who abstain from eggs and dairy products must carefully plan combinations of protein foods to make sure they get enough essential amino acids. There are many authoritative books and pamphlets to guide you in obtaining adequate nutrition from vegetable products alone; the ones you can find in sporting goods stores and university libraries are more reliable than those found only in health food stores.

Protein should make up 10 to 20 percent of your total food intake (you being an adult skier). Increased muscle mass comes from exercise, not from extra protein. Even during hard pre-season training, skiers will use only .9 of a gram of protein for each kilogram of body weight. One

quart of skim milk, for example, provides over half of your
daily protein need.

In-Race Feeding. Feeding during cross-country ski racing is realistic, and the recreational skier will also want
nourishment while skiing. Fluid replacement is necessary.
The temperature of the fluid you drink won't change your
core temperature, but it can influence the absorption time
of any food you eat along with the drink. Sugars such as
those contained in fruit juice are valuable, and dilute solu-
tions (containing only 2 to 4 percent simple sugars) will
empty from the stomach more rapidly than higher concentrations. However, it takes about fifteen to twenty minutes
for even the simplest sugar to reach the bloodstream.

Little of the sugar you take on will be used by the
working muscles; they depend on their own stored glycogen. But the nerves, which work at a high metabolic rate
during a race, need additional glucose because they have no
glycogen reserve. Proper feeding during a ski race serves to
dampen fatigue by feeding the central nervous system
rather than the working muscle.

Water. Water should be listed first among essential
nutrients for the ski racer. During prolonged activity, the
need for water replacement arises before conscious thirst.
There is less danger to performance from drinking too
much fluid than from inadequate replacement of fluid loss.

The better acclimatized you are, the more water your
body will lose through perspiration. Because the body is
able to metabolize and store salt rapidly, skiers don't need
additional sodium chloride even when they sweat heavily.
However, potassium must be balanced by supplementation,

either in the fluid feed or in the daily diet. Most fruits, cereals, and beers are good sources of potassium. When you sweat heavily, some of the water lost will be replaced from the plasma portion of the blood, which could lead to hemoconcentration—overly concentrated blood—and a drop in cardiac output if this is allowed to continue.

Minerals and Vitamins. Minerals regulate many vital processes and are essential for bone health. Calcium, phosphorus, magnesium, and iron are the four most important minerals for athletes. Calcium abounds in milk, vegetables —especially broccoli and beans—and fruits such as oranges and grapefruit. Phosphorus is found in essentially the same foods, principally milk. Athletes who get enough calcium in their diets will automatically get enough phosphorus.

One study has shown that men on a high-protein diet lost significant quantities of calcium, which is one more reason to avoid a superhigh-protein intake.

Magnesium is found in both plant and animal foods, and athletes are in little danger of magnesium depletion unless they choose a low-calorie diet and avoid such foods as chocolate, whole wheat or rye bread, nuts, and other high-caloric goodies. Dietary magnesium is important for endurance and recovery. You should get at least 8 milligrams per kilogram of body weight daily, along with adequate potassium, salt, and vitamin C. If you're in danger of magnesium depletion, good old milk of magnesia in small doses—much smaller than needed for its primary purpose— can right the balance.

Iron, of course, is essential to the red blood cells, which are the body's oxygen and carbon dioxide transport mechanism. Although the normal diet usually contains adequate iron, athletes should take special care to eat iron-rich foods: eggs, meat, green vegetables, and whole-grain or enriched cereal and flour products. Women skiers shouldn't be criticized for supplementing their diets with iron during the training season to compensate for menstrual losses of red blood cells, nor for the fact that their hemoglobin values are normally lower than men's. As many as one out of every five women ski racers may have clinically low iron levels. All racers, men and women, should have their hemoglobin and serum iron values checked once or twice yearly.

High on the list of the body's needs are the coenzymes known as vitamins. Vitamins do not in themselves yield energy or serve as building units, as other nutrients do, yet they are essential substances, triggering and regulating many metabolic processes. Only minute amounts of vitamins are necessary. The important vitamins that we know about have been analyzed chemically; they can be measured, standardized, and manufactured synthetically.

Except in cases of vitamin deficiency, which are rare in the United States, it is both cheaper and safer to get your vitamins from the food market than from the drug counter. Two of the most common vitamins, A and D, are fat-soluble, and when taken in excess, cannot be excreted through the kidneys. Children have suffered irreversible kidney and liver damage because their parents gave them massive quantities of the fat-soluble vitamins.

The B group of vitamins and vitamin C are water-soluble. Excesses of these vitamins over the body's immediate needs are usually excreted by the kidneys. In this age of hypervitaminosis, the gullible American public sends large sums of money spent on vitamin supplements down the drain, both figuratively and literally.

If a skier in training needs extra quantities of a vitamin, it would be one of the B group: thiamine, riboflavin, niacin, folacin, B_6, and B_{12}. Healthy amounts of potatoes, apples, leafy vegetables, milk, eggs, liver or other lean meat, and whole-grain cereals or bread, however, will practically assure an adequate intake of B vitamins. Niacin taken in excess can inhibit the uptake of fatty acids by cardiac muscle during exercise, which could damage cross-country skiing performance.

High levels of vitamin C intake have not been shown to have a significant effect on performance, have given no greater protection against capillary rupture, and have not decreased susceptibility to upper respiratory infections. In fact, vitamin C supplementation may increase the biochemical reactions in the body that destroy vitamin C. Human subjects in one study who consumed 5 grams of vitamin C daily had no higher blood levels than those of control subjects on similar diets without supplemental vitamin C. Claims of better performance with vitamin supplements may be a form of the well-known placebo effect: that is, it will work if you believe in it.

Vitamin E is fat-soluble and widely used as a supplement. Although it has proved to be toxic in some animals, no case of vitamin E toxicity has been confirmed in humans. However, vitamin E is probably stored like other fat-soluble vitamins, A and D, that are toxic to humans when taken in excess. To date only one Russian study indicated that vitamin E supplementation improves athletic performance, while a whole wheelbarrow full of evidence seems to show no beneficial effect from vitamin E or any other form of wheat germ oil.

On the basis of this information about carbohydrates,

fats, protein, water, minerals, and vitamins, we can advance some concepts pertinent to the cross-country skier. At present there is no sound evidence that athletic performance can be improved by modifying a basically sound diet. Furthermore, a nutritious diet can be obtained in many different ways. The best diet for one athlete is unlikely to be the best diet for all; we differ individually not only in our sense of taste but also in our enzyme systems for digestion and absorption. Conditioning and skill are infinitely more important than diet, if that diet is nutritionally sound.

Nutrition is still an important consideration for athletes, however. Psychological as well as physiological factors affect performance in all athletic events, and there is no way to evaluate the psychological importance of a certain diet. When ego and prestige factors enter the picture, science may fade into the background. And although we may not be able to modify a sound diet to improve performance, an athlete can deteriorate rapidly with a less-than-optimum diet.

The timing of eating may be as important as what is eaten. For instance, at the end of a hard workout, the stomach is in no shape to receive food for *at least* forty-five minutes. Absorption and digestion of food can be slowed or stopped by emotional reactions to competition. Therefore, precompetition feeding should consist of food each athlete knows will dampen hunger but will not lie in the stomach like a ten-pound dumbbell.

During competition, the fuel for muscular effort will come from food eaten in the previous twenty-four to forty-eight hours. Therefore, the prerace meal has three objects: (1) to dampen hunger pains, (2) to empty quickly from the stomach, and (3) to provide some energy to replace what will be used in the coming race. Concerning (1), protein will be best, and concerning (3), replacement of energy for the next race or workout is an important objective of good sports nutrition that is frequently overlooked. Average emptying times of various foods follow—although remember that emotional states can either speed or delay them:

Meats. Beef remains in the stomach about 2½ hours, whether rare, medium, or well done. Ground beef has the same nutritional value as filet mignon. Lamb stays about the same length of time. Veal, which is leaner, may clear the stomach more quickly. Pork remains considerably longer; fish and fowl, less long. Liver stays in the stomach six hours; ham, eight hours; sweetbreads or sausages, including hot dogs, will outstay ham.

Eggs. Whether poached, baked, boiled, shirred, or in an omelet, eggs generally travel faster than meat. Scrambled eggs, however, linger longer.

Vegetables. Peas, carrots, and green beans stay in two to 2½ hours. Others remain longer. Potatoes take the same time whether they're baked, boiled, mashed or whipped.

Desserts. Cooked fruits travel faster than fresh, and fruits generally empty in about the same length of time as vegetables. Most cakes, pies, puddings, and ice cream clear in 2½ to three hours. Custards and very rich desserts take longer. Pastries, especially if they're made with whole-grain flour and other wholesome ingredients like butter, honey, fruits, and nuts, are an excellent source of carbohydrates and fats and shouldn't be banned from the training diet. Ditto for wholesome candy.

Breads. Toast empties faster than soft bread because it

is broken up to a greater degree by chewing. Average emptying time is about 2½ hours.

Beverages. Coffee and tea have no effect on stomach emptying time. Cocoa and chocolate milk appear to delay it. Caffeine has been found to stimulate fat utilization, thereby prolonging the use of glycogen stores during endurance events. A cup of coffee contains about 100 to 150 milligrams of caffeine; cola, tea, and hot chocolate contain smaller amounts.

Art Dickinson, trainer for the U.S. Ski Team (USST), included small amounts of caffeine in the in-race feeds for the USST during the 1976 skiing season, including the XII Olympic Games. His impression was that it lessened fatigue. Subsequent research at the University of Colorado Sportsmedicine and Sports Nutrition Laboratory showed that not only did caffeine make athletes feel less tired, it also speeded the stomach emptying rate of fluid, glucose, and electrolytes. This action appears to be a result of caffeine's close association with theophylline, so tea might well produce the same effect.

For maximum benefit, caffeine should be taken an hour before racing and periodically during longer races. People vary widely in their response to caffeine, as to other stimulants, and it is definitely not for everyone. Milk clears the stomach slowly and is not recommended for prerace or in-race feeding.

The prerace meal should not be high in carbohydrate. Sudden flooding of the system with carbohydrate can cause a rise in blood sugar (glucose) that evokes an insulin response and a consequent sharp lowering of available energy fuel.

Carbohydrate Loading

Much has been written about carbohydrate "loading" as a technique for increasing energy. It is possible to increase temporarily the amount of glycogen by a very intensive workout when the athlete is eating a normal mixed diet, and when the athlete then switches to a high-carbohydrate diet, a "supercompensation" of muscle glycogen occurs—the muscle will increase its carbohydrate stores from about 1.5 grams to 3.0 grams per 100 grams of muscle.

If, after glycogen depletion, the athlete switches to a high-fat, high-protein diet for two days *before* starting a high-carbohydrate diet, the supercompensation will be even more striking. Muscle glycogen storage may rise to 3.5 grams per 100 grams of muscle or more (see Figure 1).

Some form of carbohydrate loading has gone on formally or informally for years. It can be valuable for skiers in

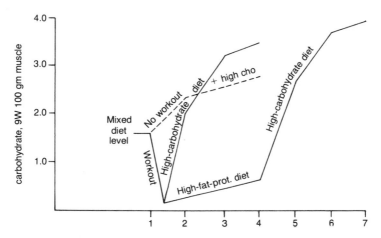

figure 1 Effect of carbohydrate loading, with and without high-fat, high-protein dietary interval.

races that last longer than an hour, but the procedure involves a loss of training time. After the intensive workout that depletes muscle glycogen, work must be light, to allow glycogen to be stored again in large amounts. Continuing heavy training would only continue the depleted glycogen level. If, after the intensive workout, a high-fat and high-protein diet is eaten for two days before you switch to a high-carbohydrate diet in order to gain the maximum supercompensation, then you sacrifice at least two training days. Many sportsmedicine authorities believe that the value of extra loading added by the two-day high-fat and high-protein diet is not worth the sacrifice of additional training time.

Control of Body Weight

Ski racers have little trouble maintaining ideal weight. The average percentage of body fat for active young women is 14 to 25 percent, and for men, 10 to 16 percent. The national ski team averages are 17 percent fat for women and 8 percent fat for men. Some women long-distance runners have been measured at 6 to 10 percent body fat, which seems a little stringent. The "average" athlete needs about 10 calories per pound just to maintain present body weight. The following formula shows the important relationships influencing body weight:

$$\begin{array}{c}\text{Food} \\ \text{Intake}\end{array} = \begin{array}{c}\text{Work} \\ \text{Output} \\ (\textit{Training} \\ \textit{and daily} \\ \textit{activity})\end{array} + \begin{array}{c}\text{Heat} \\ \text{Production} \\ (\textit{Resting} \\ \textit{metabolic} \\ \textit{cost})\end{array} + \begin{array}{c}\text{Energy} \\ \text{Storage}\end{array}$$

Whenever the number of calories eaten is greater than the calories of energy expended for basal metabolic needs plus daily work, activity, or sports training, the remaining calories will be stored in the form of fat. Whenever fewer calories are eaten than are expended, the deficit will be supplied through mobilization of free fatty acids from the fat repository areas of the body. One pound of fat is equal to 3500 calories.

Suppose a fat exercise physiologist wanted to lose weight. His food intake is 2400 calories daily; his resting needs are 1100 calories and his daily activity requires another 1300 calories. If he cuts out dessert for 7 days (at 250 calories per dessert) and adds a 20-minute jog (at 250 calories per session), he will go into negative energy balance in the amount of 500 calories per day, or 3500 calories—1 pound—in a week:

Intake =	Expenditure	Intake	=	Expenditure	From Stored Fat
2400	1300 + 1100 + 0	2400 − 250		1300 + 250	+1100 − 500

The caloric value of food, then, is the determinant of weight gain or loss. Someone eating 3000 calories' worth of lettuce who needs only 2400 calories for energy expenditure will gain weight as surely as if he or she had eaten those 3000 calories in French pastry.

Remember, too, that although good nutrition is important to sports performance, dietary deficiencies are rare in United States athletes. Any subpar performance attributable to nutrition usually results from an athlete's deviating from a normal, balanced diet.

three

NORDIC SPORTS MEDICINE

In this section we will discuss the injuries and conditions that can disable cross-country skiers, tell you how they can best be avoided, and also tell you how to treat them if they should happen despite your best efforts. The section ends with a brief discussion of the structure of Nordic skiing in the United States.

7.
preventing
Nordic
skiing
injuries

SKIING, EITHER Alpine (downhill) or Nordic (cross-country), did not become popular in the United States until after the 1932 Olympics at Lake Placid. Both forms of the sport have attracted enthusiastic participants since then, and by the time of the 1980 Winter Olympic Games, there will be more than 3 million cross-country skiers and more than 6 million Alpine skiers in the United States.

Alpine skiing injuries have been well studied. Estimates of the rate of injury, based on the National Ski Patrol System accident reports and the reports of "on-the-slope" mini-medical centers, range from 3.4 to 7.4 per 1,000 skier-days.[1, 2] If we include injured skiers who return home under their own power and seek medical advice at a later date, a more realistic injury rate of 10 per 1,000 skier-days, or 1 percent, may be hazarded for Alpine skiing.[3]

As the popularity of Nordic skiing increases, so will the injury rate, but it will probably remain difficult to estimate the rate of injury for cross-country skiers on anything like the same basis. Most cross-country skiing is not done at centers; it is informal, done at odd moments and for varying periods. The "skier-day" has less meaning as a basis for computing injury rates. A rate of 1.5 to 2 per 1,000 skier-days has been reported.[4] Scandinavian studies have estimated relative incidences as 71 percent Alpine to 29 percent Nordic[5] and 87 percent Alpine to 13 percent Nordic.[6]

Cross-country skiing is thought to be "safe," and downhill skiing "dangerous," by the general public, and many people take up ski touring because of its presumed safety. However, severe injuries have been reported in cross-country skiers, many of them heretofore thought peculiar to Alpine skiing, such as a fractured femur, a fractured hip, and a posterior hip dislocation.[7] Since the Fiberglas revolution (roughly since the 1976 Innsbruck Olympics), cross-country skiers have been going faster, sometimes as fast as 45 to 50 miles per hour on downhill slopes.[8] It is interesting that most cross-country skiing injuries occur when skiers go downhill. None of the severe injuries mentioned above was incurred on the flat or on uphill slopes.

David Hodgdon of the National Ski Patrol System analyzed 283 Nordic skiing injuries occurring between 1973 and 1978.[9] Injury rates cannot be determined, because we have no way of ascertaining the numbers of injuries not seen by the National Ski Patrol System. However, we can estimate the relative frequency of various types of injury. In this study, 27 of the 283 injuries were frostbite and 31 were exhaustion and hypothermia. A rate of 2 in 90 were found to be injuries related to a cold environment.

Cross-country skiing has been described as a sport in which upper-extremity injuries predominate, but studies show 26 percent upper-extremity and 38 percent lower-extremity injuries.[4] Similarly, in the National Ski Patrol System series there were 30 percent upper extremity and 36 percent lower extremity.[9]

Mechanisms of injury are similar for cross-country and downhill skiing; people are injured in collisions with other objects (rarely other skiers) and in falls. By far the most common fall is the external rotation-abduction fall (Figures 1 and 2).[3]

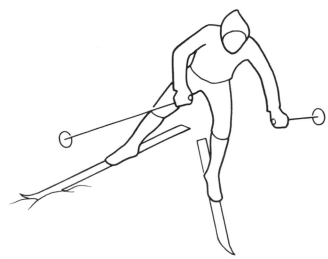

figure 1 Fixation. Inner tip of right ski caught in snow. Weight shifts to left leg as momentum carries skier downhill. Tip of right ski turns outward, causing external rotation and abduction of leg with extension of ankle.

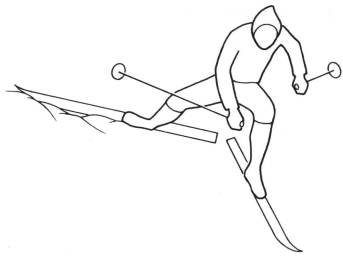

figure 2 Enchantment. External rotation, abduction, and extension magnified by leverage of ski.

The forward fall is also common but does not produce "boot-top fractures," because cross-country ski boots are not fixed at the heel (Figure 3). When the skis cross, an internal rotation fall may result. Crossed skis usually result in a forward fall, but if the skier sits back, internal rotation injuries can occur. A complete description of the wide variety of possible injuries in cross-country skiing is not possible, but several injury situations are worth mention.

Potential Injury Situations in Cross-Country Skiing

As night skiing increases, more corneal abrasions are being observed. They occur when the skier strikes unseen frozen tree branches; prevention consists in wearing goggles for night skiing.

Thumbs deserve particular attention because they are

often injured in cross-country skiing. There is no satisfactory way to ski cross-country without a pole strap, and the strap predisposes one to "gamekeeper's thumb"—perhaps more appropriately labeled "skier's thumb." When a skier falls on the outstretched pole-bearing hand, the usual strap grip prevents the pole from falling free. The strap entraps the thumb and allows the thickness and leverage of the pole to stress the metacarpo-phalangeal joint. The result can be injury to the ulnar collateral ligament of the thumb, or a fracture, or dislocation of the first metacarpal, which can be quite serious. If the ulnar collateral ligament is completely torn (Figure 4), the ligament ends may be separated by the adductor tendon, which prevents healing of the ligament. The result will be an unstable joint, causing considerable disability if it is not repaired. For example, writing may be significantly impaired because the thumb cannot be

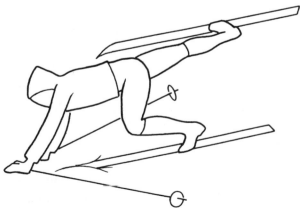

figure 3 Forward fall resulting from crossed skis.

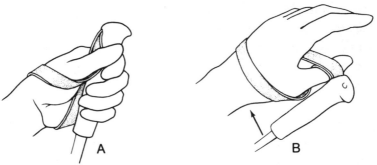

figure 4 Incorrect placement of the thumb through the strap of the ski pole can result in a trapping of the thumb if the pole is pulled away from the hand and in a tearing of the ligament on the inside of the thumb.

firmly opposed to the index finger. Surgery is recommended for these injuries.

"Skier's thumb" may be the most common cross-country ski injury. Many people seek medical advice late, and few consult ski patrols or ski clinics for this problem. But there is a wide variety of other upper-extremity injuries. Shoulder dislocations are commonly caused by catching a pole basket on downhill slopes, producing violent abduction by external rotation forces.

Ankle and knee injuries are the most commonly reported joint injuries in cross-country skiing. Ankle and knee injuries made up 55 percent of the joint injuries reported in the National Ski Patrol System data.[9] The ankle is an inherently stable joint. Cross-country equipment provides for maximum ankle motion, with essentially no external support, in contrast to Alpine equipment, which provides rigid ankle support.

The knee joint is complex, and many physicians have difficulty making accurate diagnoses of knee injuries. Knee injuries probably account for the greatest disability and morbidity because of delayed or "missed" diagnosis. The most common knee injury is sprain of the medial collateral ligament. Like all sprains, this injury is graded from I to III: mild, moderate, or severe. Most sprains are Grade I and respond to local application of ice, compression, and elevation for a limited time. Grade II and III injuries require immobilization and sometimes surgery.

Muscle strains are relatively uncommon in cross-country skiers because they seldom use maximum bursts of power. Beware of strains during dry-land training, however. If you run, you probably know that runners are plagued by a plethora of foot and other overuse syndromes, including shin splints, tendinitis, and stress fractures. Cross-country skiing uses a much smoother, more fluid motion; it can be a relief to get back on snow. For this reason, cross-country skiing is an appropriate exercise for the elderly and for many arthritics. The relatively low incidence of injury makes it particularly attractive.

There are many more types of cross-country skiing injuries in general, and knee injuries in particular, that could be described here, but this is not a medical text. One comment on equipment is appropriate. I would discourage the use of heel-fixation devices for touring skis or extra cable hooks to fix the heel. These greatly increase the potential for injury. Cross-country skiers should try to perfect cross-country technique, including steps, turns, telemark turns, and turning with the weight back. Transferring Alpine techniques, such as heel fixation, to cross-country skiing will only transfer the Alpine injury rate.

Other Common Medical Problems

Since world-class Nordic ski races are unquestionably won over considerable distances by a matter of seconds, the slightest illness can be a win-or-lose matter. What are the common medical problems that can dull one's competitive advantage?

According to the health records of the U.S. Ski Team, respiratory diseases account for more days lost from training or competition than any other illness.

Three factors are involved in the acquisition of an infection: the extent of exposure, the virulence of the organism, and the resistance of the host. The third is most significant, since you doubtless avoid unnecessary exposure, and human beings have no control over the second.

Probably through chronic stress-medicated increases of the hormone cortisol, highly trained endurance athletes have reduced immunity to infections. They become a ready target for even low-virulence respiratory organisms. Also, they may have no immediate opportunity to change from wet clothes, which alters their thermoregulatory mechanism and increases their susceptibility. Mucous membranes may be damaged by the often very cold, dry air from which ski racers extract their oxygen.

Physicians' usual admonitions, such as to spend a few days in bed, drink lots of fluid, and the common cold will subside, are unacceptable to athletes. When there is no fever, a simple coryza (common cold), with runny nose and congested sinuses, is merely an allergic response to the virus. Someone in this condition can take a good run, plunge into a hot shower or sauna, and feel splendid.

If an athlete feels ill at this stage, however, antihistamines may be helpful in relieving his symptoms, although care must be taken because of their soporific effects. As you continue to train with a cold, it may enter a secondary stage wherein bacteria that are normally present in the nose and throat take over because the virus has lowered your resistance. When fever that accompanies bacterial superinfection begins, the antihistamines are no longer useful. That is the time to see a physician for possible antibiotics therapy.

Women's Unique Health Problems. Because ski clothes may be made of artificial fibers that do not allow adequate ventilation of the crotch, women skiers are susceptible to monilial infection. Don't ignore a vaginal infection; it is easily treated with suppositories or with vaginal cream that can be used both in the vagina and on the labia, if you catch it early. Neglected monilial infections can progress uncomfortably and become complicated by other organisms less easy to eliminate.

A common problem of highly trained women athletes is amenorrhea, or absent menstruation. It may be the result of chronic stress on the hypothalamus (the part of the brain that regulates the menstrual cycle). If this happens to you, see your doctor. Most likely you will be reassured that this change will not affect your reproductive capability. Menses will ordinarily return to their usual schedule when heavy training ceases.

Other Problems. Exercise-induced asthma is common in ski racers because of extreme exertion in cold air. Symptoms range from a tight cough for a few minutes after a race to a disabling, audible wheeze that can be heard before the skier comes in sight. The athlete and his or her physician must learn the combination of drugs that works best for each suffering individual. Recent research has shown that conditioning exercise can improve exercise-induced asthma, which should be most gratifying, especially to athletically inclined youngsters.[10]

Eye health problems for Nordic skiers fall into the two

main categories of poor *dynamic visual acuity* and excessive exposure of the eyes to the sun. Dynamic visual acuity refers to the eye's ability to see clearly an object moving relative to the skier. This visual skill applies equally to driving a motor vehicle. On any terrain, dynamic visual acuity is needed by skiers to scan the track ahead for obstructions, changes in terrain, and changes in direction. Dynamic visual acuity can be affected by an uncorrected refractive error, steamed glasses or goggles, or snow in the eyes or on the lenses. Inability to see perfectly can, of course, result in injury. Skiers who need corrective lenses should probably wear contact lenses because they are least likely to be affected by steam or snow.

Excessive light is a problem, especially at high elevations and on clear days. The snow reflects ultraviolet light rather than absorbing it, and this radiation consequently hits the eyes from two directions. Ultraviolet keratitis (inflammation of the cornea), snow blindness, and poor contrast vision may result from excessive sunlight. Dark gray lenses with as high a rating for light reduction as possible are recommended in goggles.

Health Requirements

Little is required in health monitoring for the younger trail skier in good health, beyond a basic understanding of dealing with the outdoors with respect to clothing, time of day, and weather. Skiers over forty should have an annual physical examination to uncover any asymptomatic disease, since they may be placing unusual demands on their bodies for which they may be inadequately prepared.

If you are going in for mountaineering, which includes everyone who climbs or explores steadily on skis in winter weather for four or five hours or more, or for racing, you should have a thorough examination by a physician who understands the stress of these activities, and some tests of your strength and endurance. Thousands of you are now skiing for conditioning, as well as in races. Many of you are runners living in the snow belt who put away your running shoes in the winter, buy "skinny skis," and keep right on doing much the same thing you did in the summer. Your health requirements remain the same as they were for running and foot racing. For people less than forty years of age, who have no symptoms and no previous cardiorespiratory or circulatory disease, a physical evaluation may be unnecessary. A Graded Exercise Test is advisable for persons who are older than forty or who have a known significant health problem. Your physician can advise you how to obtain this test.

If, as a serious skier, you want to stay healthy and avoid injury through the winter, in addition to avoiding smoking, taking proper nutrition, and getting plenty of rest, you must stay fit. For adults, this means training three to five times a week at 60 to 90 percent of your maximum heart rate or 50 to 85 percent of your maximum oxygen intake. If you cannot obtain a stress test to determine your maximum heart rate or oxygen intake, you can approximate your average training heart rate from this formula:

$$220 - \text{your age} \times 85\% = \text{Training (target) heart rate}$$

If your age is thirty, your target heart rate will be:
$$220 - 30 = 190; 190 \times .85 = 162$$

If your age is forty, your heart rate should be:
$$220 - 40 = 180; 180 \times .85 = 153$$

If, during your training, your pulse rate, taken at your wrist or over the carotid artery in your neck, exceeds this target figure, you should slow down or pause to rest a few minutes. If you work too far below this pulse rate consistently, however, you will not be achieving the best results from your training.

Among Olympic events, cross-country skiing can burn more calories per minute (15) and utilize more metabolic units (12 Mets) at a greater oxygen cost (42 milliliters per kilogram of body weight per minute) than any of the other forty-six events. If done modestly, it is a delightful sport requiring no more health maintenance than walking. As you become more serious, and more skilled, the sport will require a bit more than ordinary attention to your health.

References

1. Gutman, J., Weisbuch, J., Wolf, M.: Ski injuries in 1972–74. *Journal of the American Medical Association* 230:1423–1425, 1974

2. Earle, A.S., Moritz, J.R., Saviers, G.B., Gall, J.D.: Ski injuries. *Journal of the American Medical Association* 180:285–287, 1962

3. Ellison, A.: Skiing injuries. *Ciba Clinical Symposia* vol. 29. Summit, New Jersey, Ciba Pharmaceuticals Co., 1977

4. Garrick, J.G.: Epidemiology of ski injuries. *Minnesota Medicine* 54:17–21, 1971

5. Westlin, N.E.: Injuries in long-distance cross-country and downhill skiing. Orthopedic Clinics of North America 7:55–64, 1976

6. Eriksson, E.: Ski injuries in Sweden: a one-year survey. Orthopedic Clinics of North America 7:3–10, 1976

7. Lyons, J.W., Porter, R.E.: Cross-country skiing: a benign sport? *Journal of the American Medical Association* 239:334–336, 1978

8. Hall, R., Martin, P.E.: Lecture. United States Ski Team Coaches Symposium. United States Olympic Training Center, Squaw Valley, California, August 1977

9. Hodgdon, D.: Nordic ski accident data 1973–1978. Colorado Springs, Colorado: National Ski Patrol System, 1978

10. Miller, et al.: Physical training effects on exercise-induced asthma, American College of Sportsmedicine, 1978.

8.
frostbite
and
hypothermia

ALL FORMS of cross-country skiing have in common two particular potential hazards, frostbite and hypothermia. Frostbite is not often considered to be a major medical problem or even a significant health hazard, except in the military, where its potential for disability is well known. During World Wars I and II and in Korea, the Allied forces had more than 1 million cases. During World War II alone, the morbidity due to frostbite caused disabilities equivalent to the loss of one division for sixteen months.[1] Today, more civilians are exposed to frostbite and hypothermia as ever-increasing numbers of cross-country skiers take to the back country each year.

Frostbite

"Frostbite, a literal freezing of living tissue, superficial or deep, occurs whenever heat loss from a tissue is sufficient to permit ice formation."[2] The mechanism of the production of tissue injury by freezing is complex. Ice crystals form in the intracellular tissue fluid. The crystals expand, and water is drawn out of the cells into the crystals, producing cellular dehydration and a hypertonic intracellular concentration of solutes, and resulting in cell death.

Crystal expansion hinders the diffusion of nutrients to the cell from the bloodstream. Extreme cold produces vasoconstriction (the narrowing of small arterioles) and promotes the shunting of blood to the body core, both of which further decrease the peripheral blood supply and increase tissue damage. Bones, ligaments, and tendons are resistant to frostbite, while arteries and nerves are very susceptible. The damage that is done by freezing is increased by thawing, as crystals expand further. Particularly damaging is the sequence: freeze, thaw, refreeze, and thaw again.

Frostbite can be classified as *superficial* or *deep*. *Frostnip* is the most superficial kind, characterized by whitish or mottled blue-white discoloration of the skin. The skin feels firm, but the tissues beneath are soft and resilient. This condition is usually seen on the nose, ears, cheeks, or tips of fingers and toes. Treatment is easy: rewarm the body part immediately by holding a warm hand on the area until it thaws. Tuck your fingers in your armpits. If you have a warm, cooperative associate at hand, put your toes on your partner's abdomen or in his armpits. Don't rub the frostnipped part. Thawing is quick, and the area will sting and become red. Occasionally blisters or peeling will develop later.

Superficial and deep frostbite appear similar at first inspection and often cannot be differentiated until the extent of tissue loss and healing is known. Frostbite shows a waxy white or mottled bluish white appearance. The skin feels cold and hard, and touch sensation is absent, although pain is preserved in the early stages. There is no swelling. The body part appears frozen solid.

It is important to note that a body part is not very painful when completely frozen. One can walk or ski many miles on frozen feet without contributing much to the degree of injury. Knowing that one can walk on frozen feet is important, for it allows frostbitten ski mountaineers or tourers to evacuate themselves to safety.

True frostbite should be treated in the hospital. The best treatment is rapid rewarming by immersion in a whirlpool bath at between 100° and 108°F (38° to 42°C). This can be extremely painful, and narcotics may be needed. The sequence of recovery is first the return of sensation, then swelling of the part, and then possible formation of large blisters. In the case of deep frostbite, the blisters will burst after three to seven days and a *mummified eschar* will form on the part, like a large, hard, dry black scab. It will remain for three to six weeks and then slough off by itself, often revealing healthy pink tissue beneath.

Treatment after thawing consists in keeping the part sterile and giving daily cleansing whirlpool treatments to avoid infection. Deep frostbite may involve a month or more of hospitalization. Amputations are rare and are done only after the eschar, the dead soft tissue, has separated completely to reveal the remaining viable tissue, if any.

Aftereffects of deep frostbite may include excessive sweating (hyperhidrosis), extreme sensitivity to cold, loss of soft tissue pads on fingers and toes, and burning pains from nerve injuries. If rapid rewarming can be started before the part thaws spontaneously, the extent of amputations often can be minimized.

In a study of 200 cases of frostbite treated by rapid rewarming, 10.5 percent of the patients lost parts of fingers or toes, with only one major amputation. The same study cites 70 cases treated otherwise, and 50 percent of those patients lost tissue, with 18.5 percent requiring major amputations.[3]

Frostbite is a significant hazard for cross-country skiers, particularly novices. Much cross-country equipment, such as cotton warm-up suits, ventilated gloves, and thin leather boots, is sold with the availability of touring centers and groomed trails in mind. Often, however, the novice has been attracted to the sport by the chance it offers to get out into the "wilderness." Touring-center clothing is totally inadequate for back-country trips. Wool mittens with covers, wool parkas, and insulated boots with overboots and gaiters are needed.

Remember the first rule: do not thaw frostbite in the field. People can walk or ski on frozen feet, but, once thawed, the patient becomes a litter case.

Racers do not often get frostbitten, because the duration of exposure is short, usually less than three hours. Frostnip can be painful, however. One-piece synthetic stretch running suits offer a particular hazard to men because they often stretch tight over the genitalia. I have watched racers suffering rewarming agony in the locker room after a windy race at −30°C. The "fur-lined" jock combined with a nylon wind shield gives good protection.

Hypothermia

Hypothermia is the condition in which the body is unable to maintain its constant core temperature around

99°F. It may or may not be associated with frostbite. People must keep their core temperature around 99°F, on the average, for optimum function of the body's vital enzyme systems, chemical reactions, and vital organs. In order to sustain a core temperature above the temperature of the environment, we must produce heat internally. Our bodies produce heat in two ways: by chemical or metabolic work metabolism, and by physical work.

The skin is the primary sensing element for the body's thermostat in the brain. Skin temperature may vary widely with the ambient temperature. It can drop as low as 40°F before numbness sets in and its sensing function is impaired. But if core temperature drops to 94°F, the condition is serious, and below 80°F death may occur.

When skin temperature drops to 40°F, metabolism or maximum physical exercise must increase eighteenfold to provide enough heat to hold the core at 99°F. The cost of this increased physical or metabolic activity is extravagant use of body fuel, and it can be maintained only for a short time, usually less than an hour.

The body has two sources of fuel, food and its own stores. Regardless of the source, there are only three basic fuels: carbohydrate, fat, and protein (see Chapter 6), and they differ in the amount of heat they can produce. Fats yield 9 calories per gram; protein, 4 calories per gram; and carbohydrates, 3.75 calories per gram. Oxygen is required for the utilization of these fuels (oxidation). Carbohydrates require less oxygen for utilization than fats or protein. This efficiency, combined with their easy digestion and absorption, makes them a favored quick-energy fuel.

When food is inadequate and stored fuel has been exhausted, the body will consume itself. Stored carbohydrates from liver and muscle are exhausted within a matter of hours. Fat reserves are next; normally these can last for days. Then the body begins to burn protein, in the form of its own muscle tissue.

We can easily understand that to maintain core temperature in a cold environment, especially while engaging in a physical activity like skiing, greatly increased food intake is required, 4000 to 6000 calories daily. Adequate fuel intake before and during cold-weather exercise is needed to avoid hypothermia; without this increased intake in preparation, death can occur within twenty-four hours of initial cold exposure.

We maintain our core temperatures by balancing heat production and heat loss, and we vary production by varying the intensity of muscular activity. Heat loss occurs in four ways: (1) *conduction*, (2) *convection*, (3) *radiation*, and (4) *evaporation*.

Conduction loss by direct contact with the environment is usually not the main means of heat loss. Under special conditions it becomes major, however; if you get wet, and your wet clothing freezes, conduction losses may be increased as much as 240-fold.

Convection of heat from exposed areas occurs by the movement of air across the surface, and it depends on air velocity. The combined effects of cold and air velocity is the windchill factor (Figure 1). A good mnemonics for this effect is the rule of 30–30–30. A 30-mile-per-hour wind at 30°F leads to frostbite in 30 seconds.

Radiation loss is constant for a given individual and is related to one's surface area.

Windchill Equivalent Temperature

WIND VELOCITY (mph)

F°	3	4	5	6	7	8	9	10	15	20	25	35	45	50
60	60	58	56	55	54	53	51	50	48	46	44	42	41	40
55	55	53	51	49	48	47	46	45	41	38	36	34	33	32
50	50	47	45	43	42	40	38	37	33	30	28	24	23	22
45	45	42	39	37	36	34	33	32	27	23	19	16	15	13
40	40	37	34	32	30	28	26	23	20	15	11	7	5	4
35	35	32	29	26	24	22	20	18	12	7	3	−2	−4	−5
30	30	26	24	21	17	15	13	12	3	−1	−5	−13	−14	−16
25	25	21	17	15	13	10	6	3	−4	−9	−15	−20	−23	−24
20	20	15	12	8	7	3	−2	−4	−13	−18	−23	−28	−32	−33
15	15	10	5	2	−1	−5	−8	−11	−20	−24	−33	−37	−39	−40
10	10	5	0	−4	−7	−11	−14	−17	−27	−33	−38	−45	−48	−50
5	5	−1	−6	−10	−14	−17	−20	−23	−33	−39	−46	−54	−56	−58
0	0	−6	−13	−15	−18	−22	−25	−29	−40	−46	−53	−61	−64	−65
−5	−5	−12	−17	−21	−25	−29	−32	−37	−47	−53	−61	−70	−73	−75
−10	−10	−16	−23	−27	−31	−35	−39	−42	−53	−60	−68	−77	−80	−83
−15	−15	−22	−28	−33	−38	−42	−45	−48	−60	−67	−77	−85	−89	−91
−20	−20	−27	−33	−39	−43	−48	−51	−55	−67	−76	−85	−93	−98	−101
−25	−25	−33	−40	−44	−48	−53	−58	−62	−75	−83	−93	−102	−105	−110
−30	−30	−38	−45	−50	−55	−59	−63	−67	−81	−92	−100	−109	−114	−120

Evaporation is the major controllable means of heat loss. As water evaporates from the body's surface, it absorbs heat. Approximately 20 percent of human heat loss is by evaporation, two-thirds by perspiration and one-third by breathing. Keeping on wet, thin clothing promotes heat loss by evaporation.

The body has several means of reducing heat loss. Peripheral vasoconstriction in response to cold narrows the skin arteries, diverting blood and heat to the core. We also shunt blood and heat to protect our core temperature. Our arms and legs seem to have been designed to save core heat —and to produce frostbite. The arteries carrying warm blood are next to veins returning cooler blood, and this proximity, with the temperature gradient, allows heat transfer from arteries to veins, preserving core heat at the expense of the extremities. Protecting and insulating the face, head, neck, and hands, all areas of high blood flow, is a basic principle of hypothermia prevention. The old mountaineering adage, "If your feet are cold, put on your hat," has merit. To this might be added, "Keep your gloves on!"

Hypothermia is a subtle menace. In its early stages, symptoms are often mistaken for fatigue. When the core temperature begins to fall, a deadly cycle is begun that rapidly becomes irreversible and fatal. (See Table below) Judgment is impaired early; the victim is unaware and unconcerned. Numbness of the skin, shivering, and loss of muscle coordination render the victim helpless. The large leg muscles are affected late. When the victim collapses, the situation is critical. The hypothermia victim depends on his or her companions to recognize the condition and to treat it early by adding heat.

The death rate in established hypothermia may be as

Usual Results of Maintenance of Core Temperature
for Several Hours at These Levels

Core Temperature, °F	Effect
99–95	Shivering
95–90	Shivering, loss of coordination, decreased mental capacity
90–85	Muscular rigidity, stupor
85–80	Coma, decreased heart rate, lowered blood pressure
80	Death, ventricular fibrillation

high as 40 percent.[4] This rate exceeds that for diagnosed acute coronary artery disease of the heart. Of first importance in prevention is adequate food intake before and during cold-weather activity.

Another useful mnemonics is VIP: Ventilate, Insulate, Protect. Ventilate excess water from perspiration. Insulate, particularly high-blood-flow areas like the head and neck. Protect from wind and wetness with appropriate clothing. You can lessen your risks if you know your enemy, hypothermia, know your environment and its whims of weather, and know your sport.

A sudden accident, however, can attack the best-prepared skier. The worst of these is immersion. The ski tourer who goes through spring ice, at temperatures of 30° to 40°F, can survive only fifteen to thirty minutes in the water. In contrast, the ski mountaineer trapped under a dry-powder avalanche can live for more than twenty-four hours.

When early signs of hypothermia are recognized and treatment is begun early, a skier usually recovers rapidly and can continue touring. Here is what to do when the victim is clumsy, shivering, and not thinking straight:

1. Stop and take shelter.
2. Remove wet clothing from the skier, even if it requires stripping him naked at subzero temperatures, and dry his skin.
3. Insulate the victim with dry blankets or clothing, using more insulation below the waist than above it. Prewarm all insulation.
4. Add heat to the victim, preferably with hot liquids. Next best is skin-to-skin contact, for example with your own body in a sleeping bag.
5. Feed the victim warm foods, especially carbohydrates.

Here is what not to do:

1. Don't warm by open fires.
2. Don't allow smoking; nicotine is a vasoconstrictor, central as well as peripheral.
3. Don't give alcohol unless the victim can be kept in a warm shelter. Alcohol is a potent vasodilator and may increase heat loss.
4. Don't attempt to give liquids to an unconscious victim.

Treat early hypothermia promptly in the field. When confronted with an unconscious, severely hypothermic victim, evacuate as soon as possible.

Established hypothermia should be viewed as life-threatening. It has not been completely understood in the past. Hospital records have shown that hypothermia victims who died all had body temperatures of 94°F. Why 94°? Because the average clinical thermometer only reads to 94°F. Special low-reading thermometers are needed to measure lower core temperatures, and they are hard to find. So we have little information about less-than-fatal established hypothermia.

The severely hypothermic victim may appear dead on arrival, with no pulse, cold skin, and barely perceptible respiration, and in a rigid, comatose state. But this death-like appearance can be misleading. An electrocardiogram should always be taken to check for cardiac activity. Many patients have recovered completely from such a condition without brain damage or major amputations after treatment. Hypothermia decreases the oxygen needs of body tissues, much as hibernation does, and severe hypothermia is potentially reversible without serious aftereffects.

Hospital treatment is basically rapid rewarming. This may be external, by water bath,[3] or internal, by peritoneal dialysis or arteriovenous shunts.[1] Those who practice internal rewarming believe that if the skin is warmed first, peripheral vasodilation may produce rewarming shock. Warming the core first will minimize this effect. The proponents of external warming believe that rewarming shock is easily treated and that the external method is simpler and more readily available. Both methods are effective, if applied by those knowledgeable about hypothermia treatment. Because frostbite and hypothermia are often present together, my own preference is for the external, water-bath method.

It might seem to you that hypothermia is of concern only to the ski mountaineer or long-distance tourer. For the mountaineer, altitude markedly increases both the hazards and the risk of hypothermia. The vagaries of mountain weather place the day tourer at risk in the Sierras, in the

Adirondacks, and in the White Mountains—all popular wilderness areas near major metropolitan centers. Ski racers are at risk, too, despite their relatively short duration of exposure. I have discussed the problem of athlete collapse during the grueling men's 50-kilometer cross-country race with Dr. Seppo Tika, who has been in charge of the medical services at Lahti, Finland, since 1971, including those for the 1976 World Championships. Dr. Tika has observed hypothermia and hypoglycemia, which is often present in hypothermia victims, in virtually all skiers who collapse in the 50-kilometer race. At Lahti he may see ten or twenty cases of collapse during a week of races. The response to warmth, warm liquids, and intravenous glucose is usually rapid, and there have been no severe cases or deaths.

Racers have expressed considerable concern about competition at subzero (Fahrenheit) temperatures. They worry about the respiratory system. It is a common misconception that one can "frostbite the lungs." Breathing cold air does produce rhinorrhea, bronchorrhea, and increased mucus, and after exertion at low temperatures one may have an increase susceptibility to bronchial infection from common viruses and respiratory pathogens. But "lung frostbite" does not exist, and there is no evidence that permanent damage occurs.

There are no FIS (Federation Internationale du Ski, the international competitive skiing association) rules or medical guidelines for low-temperature limits to competition. During the 1978 World Championships at Lahti, at −30°C, a meeting of team physicians was called to advise the jury. No uniform decision could be reached. The Russians were willing to compete at any temperature. The

Americans and the Scandinavians believed that windchill had to be considered and that −20°C was acceptable, with no wind. The races were held at temperatures between −10°C and −20°C, without difficulty.

At the Lake Placid pre-Olympics, −20°C (−4°F) was decided upon as the lower limit of temperature, and the relays were canceled when temperatures remained below this level. During the previous two days, with temperatures ranging between −10° and −20°C, 77 cases of superficial frostbite and one case of mild hypothermia among competitors had been treated at Mount Van Hoevenberg.

References

1. Unpublished data. Arctic Medical Research Laboratory. Fairbanks, Alaska
2. Mills, W.J.: Frostbite. Chicago: *Encyclopaedia Britannica.* 15 Ed. 7:750–751, 1977
3. Mills, W.J.: Frostbite and hypothermia. *Alaska Medicine* 15:2, 27–47, 56–59, 1973
4. Gregory, R.T.: Accidental hypothermia: an Alaskan problem. *Alaska Medicine* 13:134–136, 1971

9.
who
looks out
for
Nordic
skiers?

The Structure of Nordic Skiing

THE NATIONAL governing body for Nordic skiing in the United States is the U.S. Ski Association. The USSA holds the franchise for the sanction and equality control of national and international competition within the United States from the Fédération Internationale du Ski. It is also responsible for the naming and development of Nordic officials. In addition, the USSA serves a wide range of needs for recreational ski interests.

The U.S. Ski Team is a wholly owned subsidiary of the USSA. The ski team is charged with responsibility for funding, training, and naming teams for international competition. The USST maintains a full-time administrative staff, headquartered in Park City, Utah, as well as full-time coaching staffs in each of the Nordic ski disciplines: men's and women's cross-country, jumping, and Nordic combined skiing. In addition to the national teams maintained by the U.S. Ski Team, this organization is now involved in developing talent below the national team level that will one day make up the national team. The USST is supervised by a board of trustees that determines policy and hires the respective program directors.

The U.S. Ski Team is supported by commercial and individual contributions and receives no money at all from the federal government, which makes us unique among skiing nations. The U.S. Olympic Committee contributes modestly to development-level projects. Commercial support is obtained by selling U.S. Ski Team logo and marketing rights. Individual contributions come from a direct mail program.

Funds for the ski team are received by the U.S. Ski Educational Foundation, a nonprofit organization registered with the Internal Revenue Service, contributions to which are tax-deductible.

Medical Coverage. The USST has developed a sports medicine program that is directed by the Sports Medicine Coordinating Council. The council is composed of coaches, Nordic and Alpine program directors, exercise physiologists, psychologists, orthopedic surgeons, general surgeons, specialists in biomechanics, and the directors of the Alpine and Nordic medical supervising teams. The council meets regularly, under the direction of a sports medicine coordinator, to plan and review all testing and research projects for the USST. Recently, the USST Sports Medicine Society was formed to raise money specifically for the USST's research projects. This society is open to anyone with an interest in skiing sports medicine, upon receipt of an appropriate contribution.

The medical supervisory team is a group of volunteer physicians who provide medical care for the Nordic team and medical coverage for both domestic and foreign training camps and competitions. Selected regional physicians, corresponding to the USSA divisions, provide yearly physical exams for team members as well as medical coverage for local competitions.

Nordic Ski Patrols

The entire National Ski Patrol System was founded virtually by accident. In 1936, Charles "Minnie" Dole injured himself on the Nosedive Trail, on Vermont's Mount Mansfield, and it was many hours before his companions were able to drag him to a road on an improvised toboggan. With the sport of skiing growing rapidly, and with more skiers being injured each year, Minnie Dole resolved to do something to help prevent others from suffering as he had. Dole assembled some volunteers to patrol a race on that same Nosedive Trail, and by 1938 they were formally organized as a committee of the growing National Ski Association. In 1958 this relationship ended; the NSPS is now a totally independent organization.

In the beginning, Americans saw little difference between Alpine and Nordic skiing. Both took place wherever there were hills and snow, and people who enjoyed one kind usually enjoyed the other as well. After World War II, however, skiing activity became concentrated at commercial areas with lifts, and ski patrolling came to mean almost solely Alpine patrolling. But in the late 1960s and early 1970s, the resurgence of interest in cross-country skiing as a separate sport made it necessary to recognize two separate types of patrolling. Thus, in 1974, the NSPS established the new classification of Nordic Ski Patroller and a new type of patrol, the Nordic Ski Patrol.

These patrols exist with the national organization, which currently contains ten divisions (Eastern, Pacific Northwest, etc.) and is further broken down into regions, sections, and individual patrols. At the national and divisional levels there are Nordic advisers who coordinate the activities of Nordic ski patrols.

Nordic patrollers, like their Alpine counterparts, must hold a current American Red Cross First-Aid and Emergency Care card or EMT (Emergency Medical Training) card, and must be trained in cardiopulmonary resuscitation techniques. They must pass a Nordic ski and toboggan test that includes various uphill-downhill maneuvers, and must have the ability to handle loaded toboggans. Each patroller must, within three years, take the NSPS "Circle-M" mountaineering course to prepare for extended operations in winter. Finally, patrollers are strongly encouraged to take the "Circle-A" avalanche training course and the advanced levels of both the Circle-M and the Circle-A courses so that they will be more versatile.

Nordic ski patrollers perform three basic functions: they patrol at touring areas, they accompany organized groups on extended tours, and they provide coverage at cross-country races and jumping events. Nordic patrols promote skier safety by advising skiers right on the trails and also by means of printed information.

Equipment for Nordic patrols is not standardized, since each patrol faces different problems in its area. The primary difference between Alpine and Nordic patrolling is, of course, that gravity will not always help the Nordic ski patrol bring an injured skier to a road. Patrollers must pull sleds uphill and downhill. Pulka-type sleds, with chest and waist harnesses, are currently popular among patrollers, as are commercially available folding sleds, which usually use a pair of skis to help stabilize the sled. Nordic patrollers carry with them the means to make a toboggan out of available materials, if necessary.

Currently, the greatest challenge facing Nordic patrols is preparing for the 1980 Winter Olympics at Lake Placid, New York. They must cover eleven cross-country events, held on more than 30 miles of trails, and three jumping events. Approximately fifty representatives from Nordic patrols all over the country will assist the local Mount Van Hoevenberg Nordic Patrol in this sizable task.

The equipment purchased for the Olympics is well suited for race patrolling and may become standard for this type of work: the sleds are 8-feet pulkas with integral backboards,* and they have a chest harness of Fiberglas wands on the front so they can be pulled by a skier. When the wands are removed, the sled can be pulled by a snowmobile. There are also two handlebars on the rear that allow a second skier to assist in controlling the sled or to ride along when it is being pulled by a snowmobile. When the sled is being handled by skiers, skins are usually placed on the skis to improve traction on the uphills and provide control on the downhills.

Although most evacuations use snowmobiles for the bulk of the distance, there are great advantages to sleds that can be maneuvered by human power alone. First, they can

---

* Manufactured by Erline Hegg, Togo, Minnesota.

be positioned without using large numbers of snowmobiles. Second, a snowmobile often cannot reach an injured skier without seriously damaging the racing track and interfering with the race; in high-powered international competition, this is an important consideration. The pulkas can ride on top of racing tracks, causing minimal damage. And, since all race courses must be double-tracked, if both front and rear patrollers ski in line, only one track will be blocked while an injured racer is being transported to the nearest junction where mechanical locomotion is available.

As more and more people are attracted to Nordic skiing, the need for Nordic patrols will surely grow. Touring centers will attract a larger number of skiers, and as these skiers become more experienced they will venture increasingly into the back country, presenting additional challenges for Nordic patrollers. Furthermore, many cross-country skiers eventually decide to test themselves against the clock, either in informal citizens' races or in more organized races sponsored by skiing organizations and sanctioned by the USSA. For years, injuries were rare in cross-country competition, but now, with burgeoning numbers of participants and higher levels of competition, they are becoming more common (see Chapter 7).

Nordic patrols are still developing as a nationwide system capable of covering every Nordic skiing area, but the system has a solid base from which to grow to meet the dual challenges of increased recreational skiing and a larger schedule of races.

The Future

Who can tell what the future development of Nordic skiing in the United States will be? We may soon find young children in the snow belt learning to ski as early as the children in Norway—almost as soon as they can walk. Increasing numbers of young, middle-aged, and old people will become experienced skiers. And more of us will be skiing competitively as more communities hook up with the USSA. We can probably expect a greater percentage of ski-mountaineers and ski jumpers as well, and a growing need for health and safety information specifically geared toward serious enthusiasts of Nordic skiing.

I hope the information in this book, which represents a distillation of current sports medicine research on cross-country skiing, will be helpful to serious skiers who are sharpening their skills toward competitive levels. For those who are already competing, I hope it has provided some useful reminders, along with new research. See you on the trails.

index